Gerber®

BRINGING UP BABY

by Mrs. Dan Gerber

A Benjamin Company/Rutledge Book
Distributed by Simon & Schuster

A Benjamin Company/Rutledge Book

ISBN 0-87502-013-5
Copyright © 1972 by The Benjamin Company, Inc.
485 Madison Avenue, New York, New York 10022
All rights reserved
Prepared and produced by Rutledge Books, Inc.
Library of Congress Catalog Card Number 70-98175
Printed in the United States of America
Simultaneously published in Canada

Use of the name GERBER and of the title slogan BRINGING UP BABY is by permission of Gerber Products Company, owners of Federal Registration 597, 105 and others.

Foreword

Bringing Up Baby is an eminently useful and readable book. There is no mother who cannot benefit by the information contained in it. Even the most experienced mother will find in it imaginative ideas and suggestions that will be new to her. The subjects range from how to pick a baby-sitter to how to play with your baby. The chapter on play is thoughtful and fresh; following its suggestions will give a very pleasurable structure to the day.

The book's consistent theme is "Mother, you can do it!" You can manage to meet the challenge effectively. Mothers need this confidence. In an age when there are so many "authorities," many women feel overwhelmed and inadequate. Hearing and reading so many "experts" sometimes gives them the false impression that child rearing is an impossible task. Mothers will read this book feeling that Mrs. Gerber is "one of us," that she not only succeeded at child rearing but enjoyed it as well. And enjoyment is the book's second appeal. Not only will new mothers get the feeling that they can be adequate bringing up baby but they will also be glad to see that they can enjoy the experience as well.

The author nicely but simply shows how things happen between baby and parents. A multitude of little, meaningful happenings are taking place every day that offer endless possibilities for developing happy and rewarding relationships. Mrs. Gerber tries to show how some of these special moments can be encouraged and cultivated. For example, there is a wonderful section on lullabies. Sing to your baby, she says, often and in many ways. Talk to your baby, and she shows how and why. Laugh with him; read to him. Use all of the creative expression at your command. The author shows how this can be done in a spirit of loving pleasure. But she is never a compulsive person nervously pushing a child. She wants babies to have the best opportunities possible for emotional, mental and physical development, yet she never allows us to manipulate or exploit them.

Mrs. Gerber's lack of materialism will also find acceptance with the new generation. For example, her layette list is much simpler, more practical and less expensive than any other I have seen. With nursery equipment, toys and other such articles, she explains how to choose them carefully and even how to make, improvise, paint, repair and decorate them. She is cost-conscious. New brides and new mothers are often tempted to overbuy or secure more expensive and elaborate items than necessary. She makes clear that the giving of things is always secondary to the giving of love.

Bringing Up Baby does not forget the role of the father. The author reminds mothers that they were wives before they became mothers and not to turn their energies completely away from their husbands. After all, the greatest gift of all for a baby is to have two parents who love each other and then can creatively love their baby.

Robert E. Appleby, M.D., F.A.A.P.

(Editor's note: Dr. Appleby practices pediatrics in Wilton, Connecticut; he is assistant clinical professor of pediatrics at Columbia Medical School and assistant pediatrician at the Vanderbilt Clinic of Presbyterian Hospital, both of New York City.)

Contents

A Word About This Book 7

One
Nine to Get Ready 9

Two
Blessed Event! 21

Three
Getting Used to the Idea 27

Four
About Food and Feeding 35

Five
Each Day, Every Day 58

Six
Don't They Grow Fast! 74

Seven
Babyproof the Place 86

Eight
The Care and Feeding of Baby-Sitters 98

Nine
Another Word for Love 114

Ten
Play's the Thing 133

Eleven
Mishaps and Ailments 151

Twelve
Travel Is Broadening 160

Thirteen
Some Ideas 167

Fourteen
Questions Many Mothers Ask 172

Appendix—Why Throw Them Away? 185

Index 189

A Word About This Book

Even in this age of wonders undreamed of by our grandparents—an age of television, moon shots and transplant surgery—the greatest wonder of all remains that small living miracle, a baby, the brand-new human being with its very own personality and character unlike that of any other human being.

And although mothers the world over are also different in appearance, background and personality, each mother wants the very best possible future for her child. She wants to give her baby a perfect start in life by providing the best in every facet of baby care.

Today's new parents are fortunate in the help they can get, in the excellent pediatric service available, the new and wide variety of prepared baby foods, the new sturdy and comfortable baby clothes and the creative toys that are both entertaining and educational.

In only one field are modern mothers perhaps less fortunate than their grandmothers. In an earlier time when people moved around less, the young mother could turn to *her* mother, to her grandmother, aunts and her older neighbors for advice about the thousand and one small matters that concerned her baby but that seemed too trivial to merit a call to a busy doctor.

In today's highly mobile population, the young first-time mother may be clear across the United States from her relatives. She may live in an apartment building or neighborhood where she doesn't know the people who live around her or where the other women are as young and inexperienced as she is. Her teen-age baby-sitting was inadequate preparation for the full care of this precious new member of her family. And even though she reads articles in magazines advising her on proper baby care, she still longs for the comforting counsel of an older woman who has raised a family that is a credit to the community, a woman who really understands the problems that sometimes overwhelm a young mother and who is never too busy to listen, to reassure and advise her.

Countless new mothers over the past years have turned to Mrs. Dan Gerber, the mother of five and now grandmother of eighteen, reading her column in magazines and newspapers, clipping and saving them for reference and writing to her about their special problems.

Still a baby's need often has a way of being too immediate to allow a mother to take the time to write a letter and wait for an answer. And it is often inconvenient for even those mothers who save printed advice to hunt through the clippings in search for the one that may have the exact information she wants.

So Mrs. Gerber has expanded her long-standing "Bringing Up Baby" column into this book for new mothers. Here are Mrs. Gerber's experience and wisdom in her own words, in one volume, easy to understand, with an index that will help you find the answer you need easily and quickly.

Read *Bringing Up Baby* for help—and read it for pleasure.

—*The Editors*

1

Nine to Get Ready

Bringing up your baby starts well before birth—with your first hope that you are pregnant and with the selection of an obstetrician or general practitioner to guide you through pregnancy and delivery. There is increasing evidence that nutrition is important both to mother and to the baby she is carrying.

Perhaps you want the family doctor whom you know and trust or the obstetrician whom your friends and family highly recommend. But suppose you're not living in your hometown—then what do you do? Pick a likely sounding name from the Yellow Page listings of doctors?

Many young mothers-to-be write me, perplexed with this problem. I suggest contacting the American Academy of Family Physicians; the staff won't say, "Go to Dr. So-and-so," but they will give you the names of several physicians on whom you can rely. Then you can choose one with whom you feel comfortable. If you really don't like the doctor you consult, you're not obligated to continue with him. Try another, if you wish.

THE WAITING TIME

The first joy of having a baby begins when your doctor confirms your pregnancy—or even before, when you and your husband decide that you want to have a baby—and lasts until the even greater joy of the baby's arrival.

Throughout the whole nine months—or, at least, starting as soon as you tell your relatives and friends that you are pregnant—you'll get a lot of advice. Perhaps more than you need. Probably more than you can absorb. Some of it will be practical and helpful. A lot of it may be useless because it will apply to somebody else's pregnancy, somebody else's baby, not yours. Some of it may even be frightening—some friend of yours may well have had a bad experience during her pregnancy or delivery and feel the urge to tell you about it "for your own good."

As far as the medical aspects of pregnancy and birth are concerned it's wise to take everybody's advice, good or bad, with a grain of salt except that of the doctor who's taking care of you. A doctor's advice is based on wide experience and expert knowledge. Everyone else's is based on a very narrow experience, her own, and is unlikely to apply to you.

Most women find that the greater part of the nine months of pregnancy seems to fly by. There's so much to do, so many plans to make, so many things to get ready!

GETTING ORGANIZED

Of course you aren't going to spend the entire nine months getting ready for the baby—that would be unfair to your husband and unwise on your own account. But you'll find that there is a great deal of shopping and other preparations to be attended to. From a strictly practical angle, if you are like most young parents-to-be, your finances will be limited, so spreading your shopping throughout your pregnancy is a good idea. That way no purchase makes too great a dent in the budget.

The fun won't all lie in shopping. Your friends and family may be giving baby showers for you. A party is always a pleasure, and you'll receive many useful, beautiful gifts. Some favorite relative may want to buy you a special gift. To guide your own shopping and to help when friends ask you what you want for the baby, it's a good idea to make a list of things you need. That way you won't end up with six bottle warmers while some absolutely essential item is overlooked.

What *do* you need? Well, in preparing for my children and grandchildren we've found that needs can be broken down into the following categories: clothing, mealtime equipment, outing equipment, bathing equipment and nursery equipment.

Here are the lists we've made out and have found to be practical and fairly complete. Perhaps you'll want to add to them or change some of the quantities, but they will give you a good starting point.

CLOTHING

3 cotton receiving blankets
1 Acrilan, Orlon or wool blanket
3 to 6 cotton shirts
1 or 2 pairs of socks or knitted bootees
2 or 3 Acrilan or Orlon sweaters
3 dozen diapers—1 dozen if you use a diaper service
3 or 4 pairs of plastic pants
2 or 3 stretch coveralls—one-piece day and night garments
1 silk or cotton cap or bonnet
"baby bunting" or sleeping bag of warm blanket material—use indoors and/or out

MEALTIME EQUIPMENT

8-ounce nursing bottles, with nipples
4-ounce nursing bottles, with nipples, extra nipples
bottle warmer (if your doctor wants you to warm formula)
container for mixing formula, marked in ounces
sterilizer and tongs with rubber-coated grips, if your formula calls for terminal heating
feeding dish and long-handled spoon
high chair
funnel
bottle brush
nipple brush
bib

OUTING EQUIPMENT

diaper bag
baby carriage
reclining infant seat (also use indoors)
sling carrier (if you want to use one)
stroller
car bed (for later: car seat) strap, harness, seat belt

BATHING EQUIPMENT

mild soap and soap dish
baby cream or lotion
cotton pads or roll of absorbent cotton (keep covered and clean)
baby powder
safety pins (stick points in small cake of soap, keep out of baby's reach)
toothpicks (for baby's nails)
soft washcloths and towels
folding bathtub-dressing table or baby bathtub

NURSERY EQUIPMENT

pail for soiled diapers
bassinet or basket and/or crib
waterproof mattress
waterproof sheets—2 large, 3 small
3 to 6 crib sheets
playpen and pad
scales (not necessary, but you may like to have them)

That's approximately what you'll want to have. You may find that you need more of some things, less of others—for example, if you use a diaper service, you won't need to buy as many diapers.

WHAT TO BUY, WHERE TO BUY

Next comes the question, where to buy things for your baby? And more important, *what* to buy, when you are faced with several small garments all supposedly alike. How do you determine quality?

Where? Well, you have a wide choice there, from specialty shops to the local supermarket. (Our Gerber baby bibs, pants, shirts, etc., are available right alongside the baby foods in many groceries, making it easy to select a little garment whenever you're doing your grocery shopping.)

QUALITY COUNTS

Quality? Check the closeness of weave and the number of stitches. If the garment is knitted, as so many are, compare the rib knit. The number of wales determines the "give" in a fabric. Loosely woven or knitted garments won't stretch to fit the baby's needs as well, or may stretch too much and not return to size. The more stitches per inch, the better. Rely on name brands—well-known brands, such as Gerber and Babygro® by Kapart, will give you excellent service.

Well-made garments also shrink less. Often mothers think that their babies are outgrowing clothing when actually the clothing is shrinking. You might try a little test. For example, by the time you are doing your baby's laundry, you will probably have bought or been given a variety of shirts. Just put them in hot water, squeeze and then spread them out to dry. When they are dry, compare. Shirts that started out the same size may vary drastically! I'm proud to say that our Gerber baby clothes *are* well made and shrink very little. By the time we branched out into baby clothing, we knew what was important. We established standards of quality and made it a point to include those features that make for baby's comfort and well-being.

Other indications of the lack of quality are underarm seams which might chafe the baby's delicate skin. Look, too, for woven labels telling you size and brand.

In buying waterproof pants, remember that you'll want several sizes so that you can move up to the next size as your baby grows. Too-tight pants tear—and it surely isn't comfortable for baby to have pants put on that are so tight they tear.

Buy several sizes of socks, too, so that your baby's feet will always have plenty of room. You'll find it's a good idea to check sock size frequently to be sure the baby hasn't outgrown the ones he is wearing.

I love some of the new styles that are available nowadays. Baby clothes are much more delightful today than when my children were small. Our little plastic cobbler-apron type of bib is a special favorite of mine—and so practical, with that big pocket across the front to catch spills (it's a handy place to tuck a tissue to wipe little chins, too).

Those overalls with knees reinforced with bright contrasting patches are both cute and practical for babies who travel on hands and knees. And have you seen any of the clothes with patches in the shape of numbers or ABC's, applied upside down so that they are rightside up for the child looking down at them? Those add a new dimension to practicality and attractiveness—and the beginnings of learning alphabet and numbers, besides.

If you're able to sew—and so many young women are doing more and more sewing nowadays—there is simply no end to the delightful (and different!) clothing your youngster can have. You'll take great pleasure in making those small garments as you await your child's birth (and afterward, too). Not the least of the advantages is that you can save money by sewing instead of buying everything ready-made.

More than just clothing can be made at home. What about toys? Soft rag dolls are traditional favorites with children. When you stuff them with old nylon stockings, they're easily washable and dry rapidly, too.

But perhaps you don't sew. Do you have friends who do? Maybe you have talents in another line and can swap services. There are all sorts of ways of getting what you want without spending a lot of money. Trading is old-timey, but young people on tight budgets find it's one thing that never goes out of style.

A HOME FOR THE NEWCOMER

One of the greatest pleasures of waiting for the little newcomer's arrival is getting ready his own particular place to live. Whether the baby will have a room to himself or whether the "nursery" will be a corner of one of the other rooms in the house or apartment, he will need—more for your convenience than his—a place to himself, devoted to his sleeping, eating, bathing, dressing.

If lack of space is a problem with you, give some thought to where you will place the nursery. It should afford the baby privacy for sleeping, particularly in the evening when mom and dad will both be home—a corner of the living room is, then, not a very desirable place. How about the dining room or dinette? Can the living room furniture be rearranged to accommodate the dining table and chairs and the space they occupied be turned into a nursery? Or can you shift the furniture in your bedroom to clear nursery space in one corner and along one wall?

Whatever room or part of a room you choose as baby's own place, there's no limit to what you can do with a little imagination—and, often, very little money—to make it a very special place for the new addition to the family. If imagination fails you, take a trip to the public library and browse through home-decorating magazines for ideas.

Young mothers of my acquaintance have given me many interesting ideas for making a nursery both practical and attractive. You might like to adapt some of them to your own needs and will probably come up with inventive variations of your own—ideas have a way of multiplying once you set your mind to work!

The basics are simple: a bed for baby to sleep in, a dresser or other place to keep his clothes, a flat surface on which to dress and change him, a place to bathe him. You can buy these things—and dozens of others you may want to add to the basic list—at any department or furniture store. But you may have relatives or friends who will give or lend you items they aren't using at present. (It's wonderful what a difference a good scrubbing or a new coat of paint can make.)

Or you can add a great deal of pleasure to this waiting time—and save a great deal of money over newly bought pieces—by making the rounds of rummage sales, flea markets and auctions. By careful shopping—and carefully resisting the urge to outbid somebody else and spending more than you ought—you can get all you need and want at a fraction of the original cost. Clean up, paint up, and there you are!

ARRANGING THE NURSERY

There are just a few simple guidelines to follow when arranging the baby's nursery. The little one should have a place to himself that is clean, airy and quiet so that his sleep will be undisturbed and so that adults won't have the feeling that they must constantly tiptoe and whisper. (Actually, as you'll find out, most healthy babies, provided that they are ready to sleep, could doze off comfortably in a boiler factory, but parents and guests usually find this impossible to believe and are made uncomfortable for fear they will wake the baby if they make any noise.) Furnishings for the nursery should be simply constructed, designed to be useful—ornamental is fine, but useful is imperative—and, of course, easy to keep clean.

Many women—especially if they hope for a little daughter—enjoy preparing a dainty bassinet for the baby's first bed. A clothes basket is ideal. If you use a wooden one, it should be padded on the inside to protect the baby from slivers and splinters. Choose whatever color and fabric you like, but be certain that the material is washable. If the basket is plastic and is perfectly smooth without sharp edges, you may not need to pad it unless you want to "for pretty."

One young mother wrote to me that she made a very pretty bassinet by running washable blue ribbons in and out of the openwork weave of a pale yellow plastic basket. An ordinary bed pillow—a good, firm one, please; baby shouldn't sleep on anything too soft—makes an excellent mattress for such a bassinet. Give it a waterproof covering and use ordinary pillowcases as fitted bottom "sheets." If someone gives you a pretty, fancy baby pillow, keep it for show. Don't use it in the bassinet. Most doctors prefer for babies not to sleep with pillows under their heads.

Baby will soon outgrow a bassinet, however, and you'll need a crib. Again, an old one, repainted, will do beautifully if your budget doesn't allow a new one. You'll also need crib bumpers to protect him—babies can be pretty active by the time they reach the crib stage.

Besides a bed for baby, you will need a place to keep his clothes. A small chest of drawers is ideal. One of the old-fashioned ones with drawers on one side and hang-up space on the other is perfect. You may very well find one in the attic or basement of a relative. Given a good scrubbing, a coat of paint or a layer of one of the many attractively patterned stick-on papers, it will be as good as new.

A place to bathe baby? Again, it can be plain or fancy,

expensive or inexpensive. (Baby won't care—what he will care about, you'll find, is the bath itself. Most babies love having a bath.) If you like, you can buy—or perhaps you'll receive one as a gift—a special baby bath that has a plastic "tub" and, to let down over the tub when the bath is through, a comfortable flat surface for dressing and changing the baby. Or use a small plastic tub or your bathroom lavatory or the kitchen sink. If you use sink or lavatory, you'll feel more secure and baby will be safer if you pad the basin with a large, heavy Turkish towel before each bath.

SOME GOOD-IDEA EXTRAS

A screen is particularly useful if the baby's "nursery" is in one corner of a room that is also used for other purposes. You can buy one new or cover an old one with attractive wallpaper or stick-on paper.

A rocking chair is really wonderful when you have a baby. It's very convenient for feeding or just plain relaxing and cuddling that precious little one.

Be careful, in renovating old furniture, that you use *lead-free paint* on anything the baby might chew—and babies consider nearly everything chewable, especially when they are cutting teeth. I like to use the latex paint that dries so fast, especially since the brushes can be cleaned off in water.

For an individual touch, you might finish off your various paint jobs with a little decoration, such as primitive flower designs (the Pennsylvania Dutch "hex" signs, for example). If your husband, like so many young men, has ever put fancy striping on a car, let *him* do the decorating. Maybe racing stripes for a boy's room?

Large coffee cans and plastic ice cream containers make most attractive little wastebaskets when you cover them with attractive wallpaper. A towel rack fastened to each end of the crib, on the outside, comes in handy for holding blankets and towels. The young mother who told me about it suggests fastening it at about mattress level. She says it's really a step saver.

Another step saver: if you have a two-story house or a spreading ranch-style—or simply a large apartment—you'll find it convenient to keep diapers, etc., at several strategic locations so that you needn't run a long way when baby needs changing.

And speaking of towels, large ones make attractive and very practical bedspreads for baby's bassinet—beach towels are great bedspreads for a crib. They're so cheerful—and so easy to launder. Best of all, they don't need ironing! And, too, once outgrown as bedspreads, they can be used as towels again.

A holder of paper towels really does come in handy in a child's room, regardless of the child's age—infant to teen! So does a paper-cup dispenser.

In decorating, you may as well think ahead to the days when your child outgrows infancy, to the time he will be a toddler and then a child. Those days will come surprisingly fast!

Dark window shades will make nap time and bedtime easier before sunset on long summer days. Stick-on designs snipped from paper or glow-in-the-dark stars, snowflakes and other interesting shapes cut from fluorescent art paper and stuck onto the shades will be decorative and entertaining to your youngster.

ART FOR BABY'S SAKE

Are you tired of the usual nursery decal type of decoration—bunnies, kittens and so on? One young mother suggests framing some inexpensive prints of great art masterpieces. She points out that the Renoir and Picasso children are lovely, while Degas dancers are perfect for a little girl's room. So are some of the van Gogh flower prints. These pictures are large and colorful enough to appeal to even the smallest children, and she suggests that the paintings may well stimulate a child's interest in art by thus accustoming him to the best from infancy.

A bulletin board comes in mighty handy—you can tack up appointment cards, doctor's instructions, prescriptions and so on. Then, later on, you can put your youngster's prize works of art on the bulletin board.

A related idea is pegboard. It will be useful to you during

your child's babyhood and useful to him as he grows up. There are many ways you can use pegboard. Investigate the different types of pegs available at the hardware store—everything from the usual hooks to shelves can be hung on this kind of board. You might panel one corner of baby's room with pegboard, painted a cheerful color. (Just a word of caution—when you paint pegboard, poke something in each paint-clogged hole while the paint's still wet! The first time I painted pegboard, I waited until the paint dried only to find it's difficult to get those holes reopened once the paint is thoroughly dry.) You might also make a room divider of pegboard. It has all manner of uses.

An ordinary shoe bag with a hanger top makes a great "baby caddy" to hold all those little things you use in baby care, such as cotton, cans of powder, bottles of lotion. At home, you can hang it near the place where you bathe and change your baby. When you travel, you can take it along and hang it on a clothing hook or bar in the car. It's easy to carry into rest rooms and motels, too. In fact, you can even use some of its pockets to hold rolled clothing and diapers.

My daughters found that a metal record rack is absolutely ideal for children's oversized picture books. Each divider keeps a book neatly in place—and it helps teach children to put things where they belong by making it easy.

Japanese wind chimes hung near a window will pick up any breezes. Their silvery tinkle will make you feel cooler on those hot summer days, and are intriguing to both eyes and ears of children (adults, too!).

USE YOUR INGENUITY

Here's a tip for improvising—an example of how you can make something from next-to-nothing. Don't throw away a discarded window shade. Instead, give it a coat of blackboard paint (you'll find it at nearly any hardware or paint store) and then hang it on a suitably sized wall. Young children can spend hours writing and drawing on such a "blackboard." Besides being inexpensive and handy, it can be rolled up, out of the way, when not in use.

A grow-chart is another thing not necessary but useful and fun as part of the nursery furnishings. You'll need a long, narrow piece of heavy cardboard or wallboard or prestwood, a six-foot tape measure, a screw eye and paint (and decorations as you choose—decals work fine if you're not up to doing them freehand). Paint the board to match or contrast with the wall on which it will hang. Glue the tape measure to the board, to the left of the middle, with the lower numbers at the bottom. Screw the screw eye into the top—a convenient way to hang up the grow-chart.

When your baby has arrived, you'll paint his—or her—name and birth date at the top of the board. When the baby is young, you'll have to take down the grow-chart and lay it beside him while you measure him. Use a magic marker in an appropriate color to mark his height and the date. Later, the child will enjoy standing up against the grow-chart and having one of his parents measure him.

WHAT'S IN A NAME

About that name you'll paint at the top of the grow-chart—have you made a tentative choice yet? You'll want one girl's name and one boy's name chosen in advance—at least, most prospective parents do, although some prefer to wait for inspiration until they get their first look at the baby. If you want to choose in advance and unless you intend to name the child after one of his grandparents or to give him a family name—perhaps the mother's maiden name if the baby is a boy—go to the library and take out a book of names and their meanings.

You and your husband can have some very pleasant hours poring over it. Try out several names that take your fancy in combination with your last name to be sure you aren't choosing a name that will give other children an occasion for jokes. Jeannie Jones, for instance, is alliterative and pretty, but Jeannie Meaney will bring howls of laughter and cause your little one unnecessary problems.

Indeed, those nine months will fly!

2

Blessed Event!

You and your doctor will have worked out a tentative date on which the baby is likely to be born—but don't count on it. Babies come into the world when they are ready to, and nobody can predict that exact moment of readiness with complete accuracy.

But you will know *about* what date to expect to go to the hospital, and you'll want to be prepared. What can you do?

There are plenty of things. For example, well in advance of the expected date—so that your mind can be at ease while you are in the hospital—make whatever arrangements are necessary for help when you come home. Your helper may be your mother, a young relative, a friend, someone hired for the occasion or even your husband, taking his vacation at this important time.

And arrange, too, for the manner in which your helper will be notified about when she will be needed. On that same subject, make out a list of people to be notified when the baby arrives—complete with telephone numbers. Never mind if your husband scoffs that he has all those numbers right there in his address book. Fathers, especially brand-new, first-time fathers, get rattled on this important occasion. If your husband says he won't get rattled, just smile and give him the list anyway!

Get last-minute details over with—such as arranging the nursery or nursery corner—so that nothing has to be done when you and baby come home.

Remember that your husband will have to eat while you're gone. Unless he's a gourmet chef, stock the freezer and shelves with simple foods that he can easily cook or warm up. If the instructions on the package aren't amply clear, add notes of your own and tape them in place.

PLANNING AHEAD

Well in advance—the beginning of your ninth month is a good time—pack your bag. You'll need a robe and bedroom slippers (a kind easy to put on), a bed jacket or something to take its place—a small shawl, white or pastel, is a fine substitute—and at least two nightgowns, which should be pretty but reasonably opaque. You'll want brassieres and a sanitary belt. Comb and brush and hair spray should be packed, plus clips or rollers or whatever you need to keep your hair neat. Take along a supply of ribbons—sometimes the prettiest hairdo for new mothers is simply shiny-brushed hair tied back with a length of ribbon.

You'll want your toothbrush and toothpaste, of course, all the makeup you'll need, deodorant and perhaps a light, flower-fragrance cologne. You'll want a pen and a pencil, stationery and stamps, your address book—and the birth announcements that you'll lovingly fill out and mail after the baby is born. You'll need reading matter, too—perhaps this book plus some light reading to keep you amused.

There will also be things that your husband will have to bring you before you come home from the hospital, and these should be gathered together and packed well ahead of time. Your doctor or his nurse will tell you what they are— if not, ask him—but they will be things to bring the baby home in, such as diapers, a shirt, a kimono or gown, a blanket or two, a bonnet or some other head covering; in cold weather a bunting will be needed.

Unless the hospital in which you'll have your baby is on

a route that you regularly travel, make two practice runs—by day and by night—so that your husband is absolutely sure he knows how to get there. (Statistics tell us that just as many babies are born in the daytime as at night, but labor for some women *does* begin at 3 A.M., so it's well to be prepared!) Explore some alternate routes, too, in case a part of the street or road is under repair. If you plan to get to the hospital by some means other than your husband's driving you there in the car, make all those arrangements in detail well in advance of the time you expect your baby. If your husband travels, be sure someone else is lined up to take you to the hospital in case he is out of town.

So, you're ready. Admittedly, time goes slowly now. At first, time flew by—there seemed to be so much to do, so many plans to make and things to do. But now these last couple of months and particularly the last two or three weeks seem to drag by. Won't the day *ever* come?

Yes, it will—and at last it does.

THE GREAT DAY

I'm not going to talk about labor and delivery, about what happens from the moment you first suspect the baby is going to come until the time when—in triumph—you deliver him. Your doctor will give you that information, and he is much more capable of it than I am—and familiar with your particular case.

So I won't touch on the physical aspects of birth. But I'd like to say a little about what I suppose we could call the spiritual aspects. What birth will mean to you, and to your baby.

Think about this: being born must be a great shock to a baby. He has spent a long time in a warm, dark, enclosed space. He moves about, but his movements are restrained. He hears nothing except, perhaps, the rhythm of your beating heart.

Then, one day, he bursts into a different environment entirely. It is cooler, for one thing—although the delivery room is warm, it is many degrees cooler than his comfortable resting place inside you. He is held upside down for a moment to drain the mucus from his nose and throat. Then he is laid on your abdomen, and the last physical link with the place where he spent nine months becoming a human being is severed—the umbilical cord is cut. He is cleaned off, and drops are put into his eyes. And he is ready to start life.

A NEW WORLD

Think what it must be like. His eyes open, and he knows the beginning of sight. His ears unplug, and he knows the beginning of hearing. He draws breath, and his lungs learn about breathing, and his nose, the beginning of smelling. Hands are upon him, and he senses the beginning of touching. And we say there are no miracles!

Perhaps you'll have had a glimpse of your new baby in the delivery room. At any rate, you'll get your first good look at him a little later, when you are in your room and a nurse brings him to you.

First you'll think: "He's so small, he's so fragile!" (Soon you'll learn he's not all that fragile and you'll have no need to be afraid of handling him.) You'll think he's beautiful and your husband will agree with you, perhaps a bit doubtfully (he's not a new mother). You'll count his arms and legs, his fingers and toes, as all new mothers do, to allay that small doubt you've had, the question in your mind, "Am I a good enough human being to bring a perfect baby into the world?"

Perhaps you and your husband, with that adoring foolishness of all new parents, will decide that the baby has your pretty nose, his father's wide-set eyes—even though the truth of the matter is that all baby noses look like nothing but baby noses and all baby eyes are pretty much alike for the first few weeks, too!

A NEW WAY OF LIFE

Birth is the end of one way of life for you and your baby, the beginning of another for you both. It is a kind of separation, but in another way an even more wonderful coming together. You know that for a while—quite a long while, really—this little, suddenly living creature will be totally dependent on you, and that gives you a feeling of awe. You hold him close for the first time and know that here he is, and he is yours. Perhaps, as you cradle him in your arms, he recognizes that familiar heartbeat and is content. And so are you.

What is he like, this new baby of yours? Here we can speak only of averages, but averages say that if the baby is a boy, he will be a little heavier and larger, and grow a bit faster, than a baby girl. For the first three or four months he'll eat as if eating were going out of style tomorrow. So don't worry when, at the end of that time, his appetite decreases a little—baby is simply adjusting. If he continued to eat and grow throughout his formative years as he does those first three or four months, he would turn into an adult the weight of an elephant, the height of a giraffe!

The average full-term baby is from eighteen to twenty inches long; some big babies may measure twenty-two inches. The rule goes like this: the baby grows ten inches during his first year; he does this in a diminishing manner, adding four inches the first quarter of the year, three inches the second quarter, two inches the third quarter, one inch the final quarter. During his second year, baby's rate of growth will slow down even more. But these, don't forget, are only averages.

HOW BIG WILL HE BE?

Weights vary even more significantly than length. Full-term newborns may weigh from five to ten pounds, sometimes a bit more. During the first few days of life, most babies lose up to 10 percent of their birth weight, and then regain the loss by the tenth to twelfth day. (Coming into the world *is* a shock!) One-and-one-half to two pounds a month is the average weight gain during the first three months. By the time he is five months old, the average baby will have about doubled his birth weight. In the second six months of his first year, he will gain about a pound a month, resulting in a tripled birth weight by the end of that year. After that, the rate of gain slows down considerably. Remember, though, that these are averages. Few babies will follow these figures exactly.

What else will you wonder about when your baby is brand-new? His fontanel, perhaps, the "soft spot" in his head where the bones have not yet grown together. Is it too big?

Don't worry. It may be very small or very large or anywhere in between—all sizes are normal. When will it close? Probably by the time the baby is eighteen months old or thereabouts. Is it very delicate—are you likely to injure it? No, indeed. Nature, in her miraculous way, has provided a tough membrane covering, sturdy as heavy canvas, to protect the place until the skull grows to close it.

When will he cut his first tooth? As early as the end of his fourth month, as late as early in his second year—babies, as you can see, pay very little attention to schedules. Sometime between his sixth and ninth months, the average baby cuts his first tooth or perhaps two teeth or three. By the time he's one year old, baby may have anywhere from one tooth to ten teeth—but again, that's the average. Your baby may be different, and if he is there's nothing to worry about. Each baby has his own pace for developing because each baby is himself, different from any other.

When will he first smile at you—a real smile of love or mirth, not just a reflex action? At about two months. (By then he'll have a personality all his own, too—a social being!)

When will he be able to hold his head erect? At around four months.

When will he sit alone? Six months to nine months.

Crawl? Again, six to nine months.

Walk? Probably between twelve and fifteen months.

But now he's just newborn, and you have all the time in the world ahead of you in which to take joy in his development.

With a smile on your lips, you drop off to sleep. . . .

3

Getting Used to the Idea

Going home is fun. And yet you're a bit apprehensive, too.

These days in the hospital have been wonderful. Friends and relatives have made a fuss over you, as if you'd just managed to produce the first baby ever! You've gotten flowers and presents, and everyone has said how well you look and how absolutely beautiful the baby is. By now you're used to the idea that you're flat in front once again and that when you stand up and look down, you can see your feet. The thought of getting back into your non-maternity clothes—without any trouble, or perhaps with very little dieting?—is exciting.

But here in the hospital you've had all the experienced baby help in the world. The place swarms with nurses and doctors. After today, it's going to be up to you. You'll have to be both mother and nurse, besides housekeeper, chief cook and bottle washer. (With a baby, that's not a joke!) And you wonder: am I up to it? Can I give this precious little life entrusted to me the care he deserves? By now, there's no question about love. You can give him all the love any baby could ever need. But you're no expert. Will you face the challenge and meet it well?

You take a deep breath and vow that you'll be the mother of the year, the century. Of course you can do it!

And here comes your husband to take you and the new member of the family home.

Home, you'll find, looks good to you—very good indeed. But it can also look rather frightening. There are beds to be made, dishes to be washed, meals to be cooked, rooms to be cleaned. There were always those, of course. But now there's baby to take care of, and you know that the washing and the ironing, the cleaning and the cooking, will somehow have to be fitted into a day that centers around baby. You'll have help, probably, the first few days. But after that you and baby will be alone together all day. Are you up to it?

TAKE IT ALL IN STRIDE

Relax. Enjoy yourself. This is quite an accomplishment on your part, creating a new human being. Pregnancy and labor weren't all fun (even the adoption process has its own anxieties) but they have their rewards, too, and now that your baby has arrived, and you have brought him home, you have every right to be proud of yourself and your offspring and to enjoy him to the utmost. And a relaxed mood is beneficial to both of you.

Of course, selecting the doctor who will help you care for your baby is all-important in keeping that relaxed mood. You may prefer a family physician, especially if he delivered your baby, or you may choose a pediatrician, who specializes in baby care.

My cousin told me about a good idea: her neighbor selected a pediatrician and visited him in his office *before* her baby was born. That's very sensible. I bet she was much more relaxed and confident when she took her baby to see the doctor at his office for the first time.

You'll be wise to acquaint yourself with the resources available in your community for expectant parents and babies. So check your hospital as well as county and municipal governmental agencies. Many sponsor expectant parents classes and maintain well-baby clinics, inoculation centers and other services at nominal or no cost.

You're going to do the right things for your child. You

want to, or you wouldn't be reading this. You've probably read other baby books and magazine articles as well, and perhaps you have or will attend classes for young parents. And to back up all this up-to-the-minute knowledge, you've inherited the instincts of untold generations. No need for you to lack confidence in your ability to know what to do for your baby! You may feel clumsy, all thumbs, at first, but the baby isn't a critical judge. Your loving tenderness means far more than the experienced but necessarily limited care of the nurses at the hospital.

If you keep a scrapbook about your baby, you'll find that you'll always value it. You might save a copy of the local newspaper from the day of the baby's birth and keep it in the scrapbook. Take snapshots and make notes of the baby's antics and achievements. It's a good idea to make notes, as well, of immunization dates and the baby's height and weight at intervals. Not only will you enjoy looking at the scrapbook and remembering, in the years to come, but your child, too, as he grows up, will be interested.

If in later years he proves somewhat jealous of a new brother or sister, the scrapbook will be proof of your love and interest, and each child will enjoy seeing what he or she did as a baby. To an older child or teen-ager, the newspaper will be of great interest, including the comics and hilarious out-of-date advertisements and prices.

One thing you'll want to start soon after you're home is a list of questions to ask the doctor. Even if you tell yourself, "Oh, I'll remember everything," don't count on it. You'll come home from your first checkup at the doctor's and realize you've forgotten to ask the question you consider most important of all. So make a list—it will help to save the doctor's time and yours. You'll find that there are all sorts of questions you'll want to ask, all sorts of information you want to gather. Jot it down while you think of it—that's the safe-and-easy way.

DON'T WORRY ABOUT BABY'S SLEEP

Doesn't the baby sleep a lot! Of course, some sleep more than others, but generally speaking, for the first two months a baby sleeps most of the time that he is not being fed or bathed. He stays awake increasingly longer as he gets older, sleeping eighteen to twenty hours when two to three months old, sixteen to eighteen hours when four or five months. And from six to twelve months, the average baby sleeps twelve hours at night, with morning and afternoon naps. Each baby seems to form his own private sleeping schedule and pattern of wakefulness. Just let him, and accommodate your schedule to his. You'll both be happier and better-tempered.

In writing me, many new mothers mention their worries over whether their babies get enough sleep. No need to get upset: a baby will get the amount of sleep he needs. An active, high-voltage baby usually sleeps less than a placid baby, but there isn't any indication that the one thrives better than the other. They're just different, just as different as the adults they will someday become.

But perhaps your problem is whether *you* get enough sleep, what to do when you are ready to drop and the baby is wide awake or when baby is in one of those distressing states of being tired but fretting instead of relaxing and going to sleep.

Many young mothers have found these tricks helpful in lulling a baby to sleep: a gentle rubdown with lotion (soothing, gentle smoothing-on of the lotion, not a brisk massage, which will wake him up even more!) and a little warm milk. A few minutes devoted to rocking the baby and softly singing a lullaby is another good sleep coaxer. It needn't be a traditional lullaby; any song that you enjoy singing is fine. And many babies, once in bed, seem to prefer being tucked in cozily. After all, the baby spent nine months cuddled in close quarters before birth, so this probably gives him a feeling of friendly warmth and security.

IS IT DAY OR NIGHT?

Another idea, for the older baby who gets his days and nights mixed up: when he is awake during the evening, encourage him to stay awake. You and your husband might try playing games—count the baby's fingers and toes, for instance—and encourage mild exercise. Gently, though; no roughhousing or exciting play, since stimulation can prolong wakefulness. This may well turn into the most pleasant part of the evening! Then a bath and "bedtime snack" for your baby will help him sleep longer and more soundly. The cuddling as you feed him has a lulling effect on the baby. On you, too.

Should the baby sleep on his back or on his tummy? That's to some extent up to the baby. Some babies prefer one position, some the other. You might try both and see which one your baby likes best. When the baby sleeps on his tummy, the covers do stay put better, diapers absorb more moisture, and air bubbles come up more easily. The most sensible thing to do is to be guided by your doctor, who ought to have the final word on this subject.

Many mothers, who worry about whether their babies are sleeping enough and notice how the babies waken at the slightest sound, will try to keep the house completely silent. You'll find that this isn't necessary. In fact, it has the reverse effect: it makes the baby even more sensitive to sound. Go on about your household chores and don't worry about making a little noise. It may even be reassuring to the baby. Ever live near railroad tracks? Soon you don't notice the trains at all, and the same is true for your baby's sensitivity to noise. He gets used to everyday sounds and doesn't notice them. If you normally have a radio or television on, fine.

GET ALL THE HELP YOU CAN

Oh for the good old days! In your reading, have you encountered any of the books and articles, apparently aimed at the jet set, offering advice in selecting a good baby nurse, nanny or governess? In some fiction, it seems that such nurses are as plentiful as dandelions in April, but in real life, how many young mothers can afford them even if they could find them? You may indeed have moments of feeling utterly overwhelmed, of wishing *you* at least had a staff to run the house while you devote yourself to the baby.

In principle, the idea is sound. A new mother does not have her full strength and needs extra rest in order to do well by baby and husband. If your mother or mother-in-law, or an aunt or a cousin, has come to help out for a time after you leave the hospital, fine.

Even if you do have outside help when you first come home from the hospital, your volunteer won't want to stay forever, for she has her own life to lead. But she can lighten your load for the short time it will take for you to regain your strength. Perhaps your mother or mother-in-law lives too far away and you have no one to whom to turn. The fact remains that you need all the rest you can get for a while. Hopefully, you had enough energy during the last days of pregnancy to put your home in good order. Now is the time to "coast" for a while. Do what housekeeping you must, but when baby is sleeping, grab a quick nap yourself, especially if he has been getting you up in the night! You'll be a better wife and mother for taking care of yourself.

An associated problem is that of visitors. Of course you are proud of the baby and want to show off your living miracle to friends and relatives. But if they stay too long, your baby will be fretting and you will be exhausted. If you casually bring into the conversation that you need some rest, the visitors will understand and limit the length of their stay. If they don't take the hint, tell them politely but firmly that it is nap time.

THE KEYWORD—ORGANIZATION!

It's a good idea to organize your life to simplify your work. Luckily, in this age, there are all sorts of delicious, easy-to-fix frozen and pre-prepared convenience foods to feed the adults in the family. Oven meals are especially easy; everything just goes in and cooks without a lot of watching. You might cut down on dishwashing by using paper plates for a time. They come in many pretty patterns nowadays and can be discarded after the meal.

Don't forget that you were your husband's wife before you became the baby's mother. Try not to make the mistake of some new mothers—becoming 100 percent the baby's mother, with seemingly little time for or interest in your husband. Regardless of how thrilled he is with his child, he'll

---

Try to schedule your day so that baby's feeding times are always relaxed and unhurried. *See pages 36–37 for baby feeding tips.*

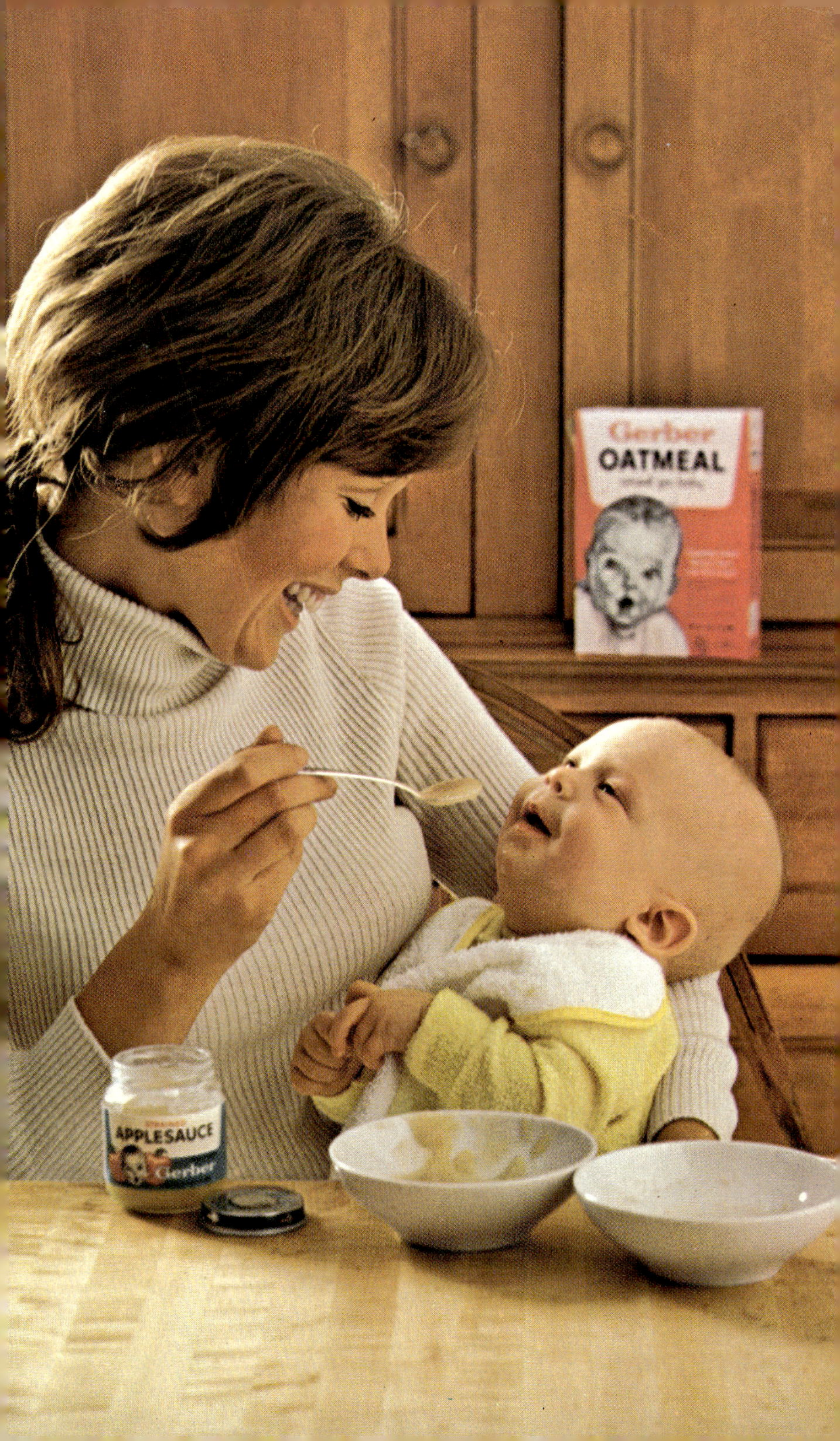
Gerber
OATMEAL
APPLESAUCE
Gerber

Most babies are given cereal as a first solid food. Strained foods soon follow. *See pages 42–43 for baby feeding tips.*

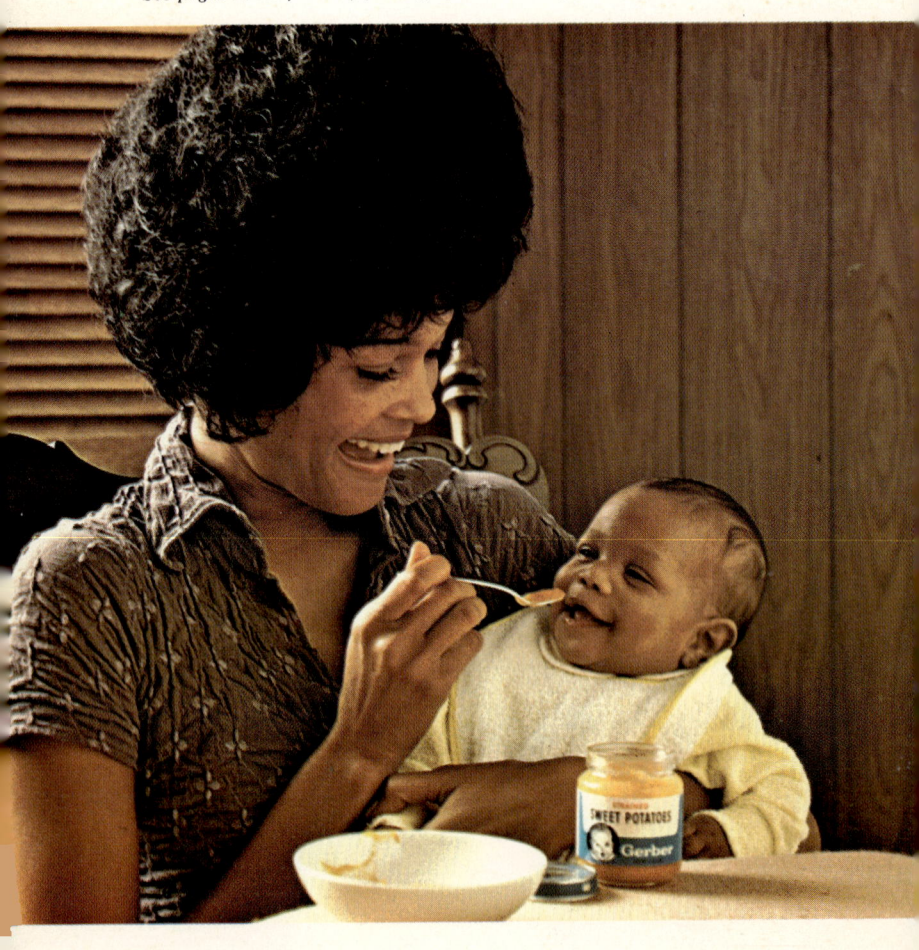

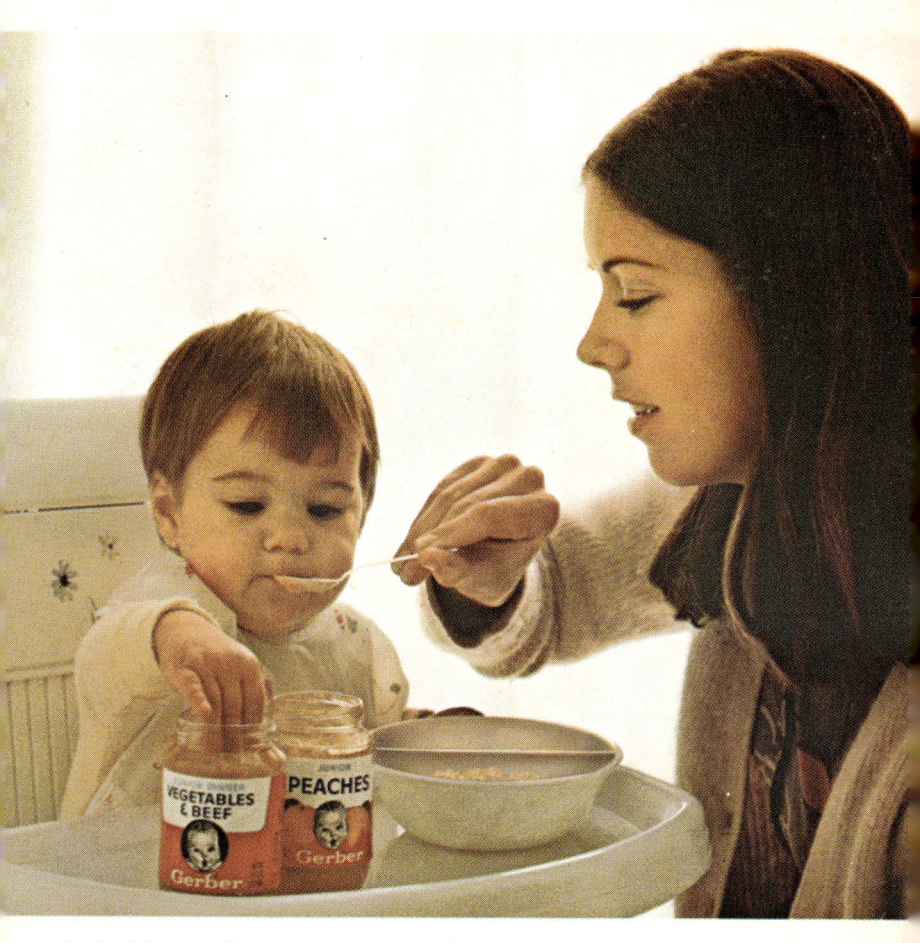

Junior Dinners, with fruit serving as dessert, are added to the diet of the slightly older baby. *See pages 48–49.*

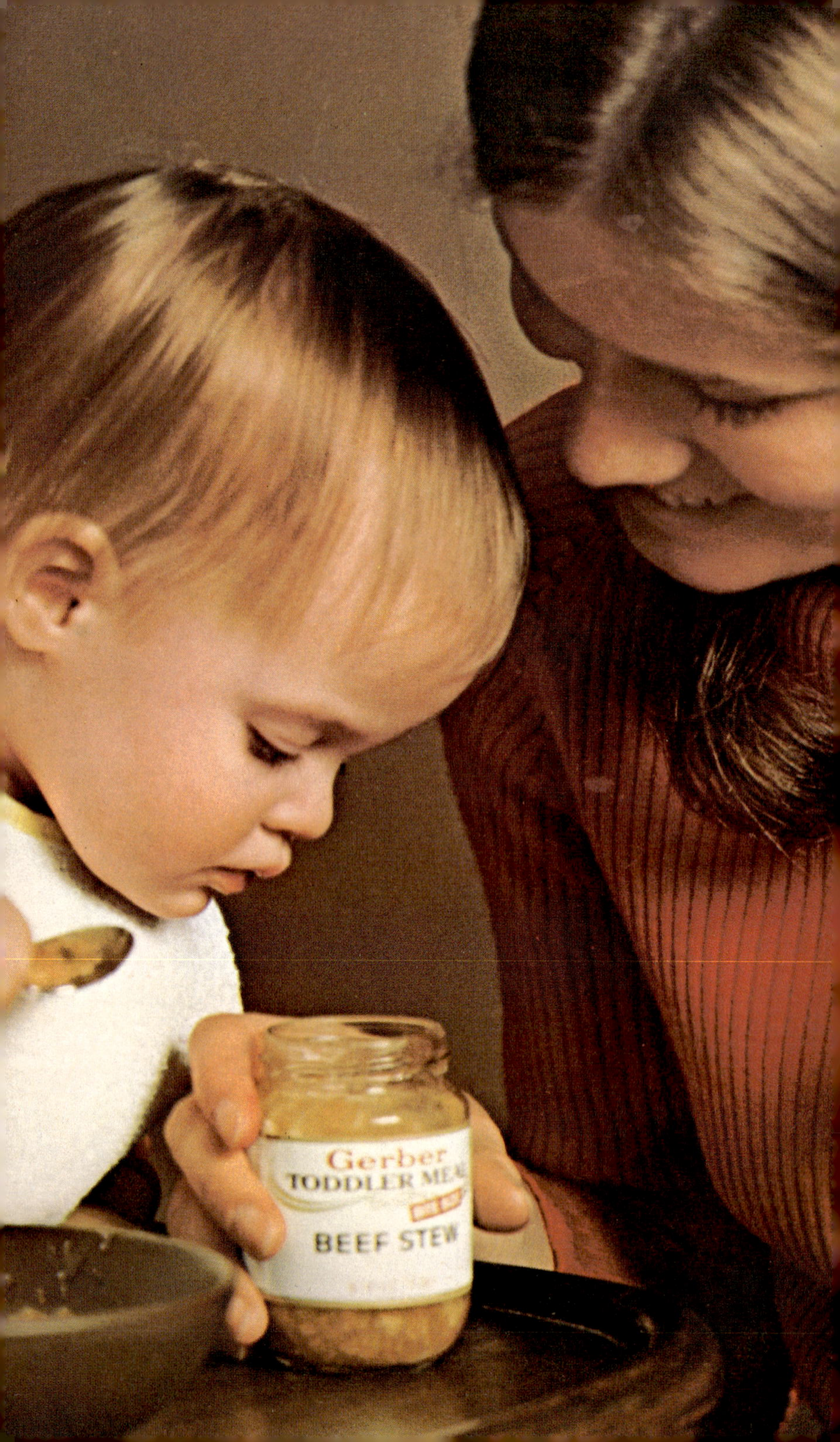
Gerber
TODDLER MEA
BEEF STEW

appreciate moments of receiving your full attention as much as he did during courtship days.

Freshen yourself up after your afternoon nap to look pretty when he gets home. Take an interest in his day. If he wants to help take care of the baby, wonderful. As with you, it doesn't matter if he feels awkward at first; the important thing is the love and protection that the baby senses. It's an established fact that babies like to be held by men! This closeness with the baby will be a great satisfaction to him and will make it truly "our" baby, not seemingly yours alone.

WHAT TO FEED HIM—AND HOW

Bottle- or breast-feeding? With rare exceptions, this should be entirely your own choice, and I suggest you don't give in to outside pressures, pro or con. Your baby will thrive equally well on either breast milk or modern formula as a basic food. At any rate your doctor will soon be prescribing supplementary foods, whichever method you choose.

Regardless of the way you feed your baby, it is important to cradle him in your arms at feeding time. Please don't leave him with a propped-up bottle! Of course if you breast-feed, you will hold and cuddle your baby, but cuddling is equally important to a bottle baby, for it gives him a feeling of contentment and security. I have also discovered that in bottle-feeding, the baby is less inclined to swallow air if he is held in an upright position while being fed. Keeping the bottle tilted so that the nipple is always filled with milk also helps prevent air swallowing. Many doctors now feel it is unnecessary to heat the formula, but if you prefer warming it and have a baby who is a "slow eater," as my son Dan, Junior, was, you might try a trick I found handy. There was no speeding him up, but slipping a knitted coaster over the bottle helped to keep it warm longer.

SUCKING IS GOOD EXERCISE

The sucking exercise a baby gets in nursing plays a great part in the development of jaw and mouth muscles, and the firmer the nipple of the bottle, the better the exercise will be. When the nipples become swollen or soft from boiling, discard them and get new ones.

When your little one is about fourteen months old, he will begin to relish the texture of Toddler Meals. *See page 54.*

You'll find, as I did, that a baby isn't hungry every time he cries. He may need to be bubbled or have his diaper changed, or he may simply be lonely. How can you tell if he *is* hungry? Well, a pretty good guide is the length of time since the last feeding. If that was only an hour or so earlier, check other factors. A certain amount of crying is a normal activity, but it is no longer considered at all advisable to leave the baby to "cry it out." This makes him feel that this is a hostile world, and it may cause him to become a belligerent, uncooperative child. Comforting an unhappy baby actually makes him a "good" baby, since pleasant experiences make him feel that this is a friendly world, which gives him increased self-confidence.

And then, sometime around the age of one to two months, the big moment will come—your baby will smile at you! Believe me, that first smile makes the 2 A.M. feedings, soiled diapers and all the rest well worthwhile. Usually you get this first real smile as you're talking to the baby while taking care of him. Then for a while you may have to coax the baby to smile, but it won't be long before your baby will break into a delighted grin each time he sees you.

4

About Food and Feeding

Although I have a great interest in nutrition and am confident that meals served in my home are nutritious, I am not technically trained in this science. Therefore I have asked a nutritionist with our company for many years, Edna Mae McIntosh, to write this chapter.

Your baby is wonderfully different—an individual unlike any other baby you have ever known or ever will know. Recognize this difference, treasure it and even cultivate it. It is what makes your baby so precious to you.

Babies may vary from the average and still be entirely normal and healthy. The best way of being certain your baby is progressing well is through regular checkups by a doctor. Your doctor will not watch weight and height gains alone. He will judge all phases of growth, development and nutritional status. He is the one to give you helpful suggestions tailored to your baby's specific needs.

Even your baby's food needs will vary from those of another baby. Size and physical development, bone structure, proportion of bone to the rest of the body, rate of growth, activity, heredity and many other conditions determine how much your baby will eat. This very important subject of your baby's diet is a matter for advice and supervision of your doctor.

HAPPY MEALTIMES

Your baby's first-year diet should be prescribed by your doctor. But you have the day in, day out responsibility of carrying out these directions. The job is larger than simply buying and feeding certain foods. It includes making every mealtime a happy time—and that can be very important.

Through happy mealtimes your baby's physical and emotional hunger are both satisfied. Since food meets a basic need, it is one of the first means by which a newborn baby can be given security. The young nursing baby, cuddled in his mother's arms, also has the warmth and support which satisfy two other basic needs. These early mealtimes are indeed happy!

Early in your baby's development, mealtimes become more than just a means to physical comfort. Your love—expressed through your voice, your smiles and gentle handling—becomes meaningful. Before long, these are as important to happy mealtimes as the food.

A little later, your baby makes many other pleasant associations with eating. He learns to like the bright color, smooth texture and pleasant odor and flavor of certain strained foods. He begins to anticipate a meal, just by being placed at his feeding table or in his high chair, having a bib tied around his neck, seeing a baby picture on a package of cereal or watching the warming of a dish of strained food. He learns to enjoy the companionship of other family members.

After a while it becomes impossible to count all the things that make your baby enjoy his meals, although his pleasure is obvious. You will feel it worth much planning and effort to maintain this happy state.

From the first feeding, you will want to see that you—not your baby—are in control of the situation. This does not have to be accomplished with a battle royal. Arguing with a tiny baby is childish and futile. Calm, gentle, pleasant and patient firmness are earmarks of maturity in parents. As expressions of your love and concern, they give your baby far more security than does having his own way.

Your baby's grandparents probably were "raised by the book." Perhaps you were too. Fortunately, the rigid feeding schedules that were insisted upon during the first forty years of this century have been abandoned. Modern parents recognize individual differences in food needs. This is true of the amount of food needed and the frequency with which it should be fed.

Most babies will set up their own schedules—a rhythm of eating and sleeping in keeping with their own special needs. "Big eaters" usually space their meals farther apart, while other babies will want less food at one time, but more frequent feedings. With a little give and take, both the baby and the rest of the family can settle down to a reasonably regular schedule. A recognition of individual differences and a calm flexible attitude toward adjustments, if they are needed, are all it takes.

CATERING TO BABY'S LIKES

Knowing the kinds of foods babies like is helpful in keeping meals pleasant. Infants instinctively accept foods that are sweet, slightly sour and slightly salty. They reject bitter foods and those strongly sour and strongly salty. The basic tastes, in combination with odors, contribute to the overall characteristic flavors of different foods. Most baby foods have flavors infants naturally like or readily learn to like.

The textures and consistencies that infants like vary with age. Newborn babies want liquids only. Within a few weeks, the "feel" of starting cereals, strained meats, vegetables and fruits becomes acceptable. Junior (minced) foods and teething biscuits are favored after the appearance of a few teeth. You can use each progressive stage to add to the total variety of foods known and accepted by your baby.

When served "warm," baby foods should be just above body temperature. More leeway is possible when serving foods "cold." Recent studies have even shown good acceptance of cold formula. Though not necessary, it is still customary to serve formulas, meats, vegetables, egg yolks, dinners and high meat dinners warm. Precooked cereals usually are mixed with warm milk. Fruit juices, fruits, cottage cheese and desserts are more appropriately served without heating.

Even in the first year, babies react to examples set by parents and older children. They are accomplished mimics at only a few months. Any attitude expressed toward food should be a pleasant one. Never indicate or discuss a food dislike in front of a baby.

A DAILY FOOD PLAN

In the interest of meeting his individual needs, your baby's diet should not be rigidly standardized. However, the first year should see a gradual transition to the following broad pattern. This means working toward including in the diet, daily, suitable portions of foods selected from each of the following groups:

Milk group, including cheese and ice cream.

Meat group, including beef, veal, pork, lamb, poultry, fish, egg (dry beans, peas and nuts are occasional alternates for older children and adults).

Vegetable-fruit group, including a dark-green or deep-yellow vegetable (for vitamin A value) and citrus fruit or other good vitamin C source, daily.

Bread-cereal group, emphasizing the whole grain, enriched or restored varieties.

This daily food plan is a practical one to follow. It's so general, it can be used for persons of all ages and in accordance with national, regional or social food patterns and individual likes and dislikes. It is a simple, flexible and enjoyable way of consuming an adequate diet without worrying about individual nutrients.

MOST BABIES START WITH MILK

Milk is the principal food of babies and plays a major role in the diets of young children, for it furnishes a wide variety of important nutrients. Whole milk contains significant amounts of vitamin A, riboflavin and thiamine. It is the best practical source of calcium and a good source of phosphorus. The proteins in milk are present in liberal amounts and are of excellent quality, well utilized in the growth of infants and children. Milk contributes many trace minerals and several of the lesser-known vitamins.

It would be difficult to argue against the "rightness" of human milk for human babies. Most mothers who wish can breast-feed, but many factors can influence this personal choice. It is well to make a tentative choice between breast- and formula-feeding well before the baby is born. Either method gets off to a better start with advance preparation.

The final decision for or against breast-feeding should be yours. Breast-feeding can be confining—you will always have to be home when baby is fed. If you are the sort of person who does not like to be regimented by a schedule, perhaps you will choose not to breast-feed your baby. If so, don't feel guilty about your choice. Remember, instead, that if you feel hemmed in by breast-feeding, chances are your baby will sense your dissatisfaction. So choose formula, but do hold and cuddle the baby while you're feeding him, except on those times when you feel you must "take off"—when you will, of course, leave a responsible mother substitute to care for your baby and to feed him in your stead.

Today, most babies can be expected to thrive on formula-feeding if that choice is made. The sanitary aspects of formula-feeding have long since been licked with sterile canned formula and good standards of food handling. Babies' nutritional and physiological needs have been well considered in the construction of modern formulas. But you still have something important to give—the love and cuddling every baby should have while nursing either bottle or breast.

Your baby's doctor should prescribe the specific formula, technique of preparation and approximate schedule for feeding. His directions will be based on your baby's own nutritional and digestive needs. He might prescribe a "from scratch" formula but is more likely to specify one of the convenient "premodified" formulas that need no diluting or only diluting with an equal amount of boiled water.

Convenience is not the only advantage of "premodified" formulas. As long as they're used, a separate vitamin preparation isn't needed—with less chance for overdosage.

In a newsletter to members, the Committee on Nutrition of the American Academy of Pediatrics has reminded them of the effectiveness of formula *with added iron* in preventing iron-deficiency anemia in infants and young children. They advocate formula *with iron* for routine prescription and its use extended over the entire first year.

Despite its nutritional excellence, plain cow's milk isn't a "perfect food." Even in the generous quantities usually fed to babies, it is decidedly deficient in iron, vitamin D and folic acid and somewhat borderline in certain other vitamins and minerals. That's why doctors recommend the introduction of "supplementary foods" before a baby's body stores of these nutrients are depleted.

DOES BABY NEED WATER?

Most of a baby's water needs are met through breast milk or formula. To supplement this, the doctor will probably tell you to offer a little water between feedings, letting the baby's thirst dictate the amount taken.

Two or three nursing bottles of water, in about four-ounce portions, should be prepared daily. One method is to pour freshly boiled water into sterilized bottles. The other is to put cold tap water into clean bottles and apply "terminal heating" (if you use that method in preparing the milk formula). Bottles of water should be kept at room temperature with sterile nipples inverted or covered. Serve the water at room temperature. After a few months, boiled and cooled water may be kept in a covered container and fed by cup.

HOW ABOUT VITAMINS

If you're breast-feeding, the doctor will probably prescribe a reliable source of vitamin D within your baby's first two weeks. If you're feeding one of the premodified, vitamin-enriched formulas, that will contain sufficient vitamin D and other necessary vitamins. If a separate vitamin D source or multivitamin preparation is prescribed, follow the doctor's directions exactly. Too much vitamin D can be dangerous.

Breast milk supplies only borderline amounts of vitamin C and cow's milk, heated for formulas, contains little. That is why most babies are started on a vitamin C supplement in the first month.

Orange juice is the traditional vitamin C supplement

for babies because it is a rich source and infants like it. Gerber strained orange juice for babies is specially processed. Its vitamin C content is uniformly high and, through pasteurization, is better retained during refrigeration than in fresh juice. Strained orange juice for babies will go through a nipple. Peel oil and seed protein, to which some babies are sensitive, have been kept to a minimum.

Gerber strained apple juice with added crystalline vitamin C is gaining favor with many doctors as the "starting" juice. Young babies accept it readily, and it seldom upsets them. Older babies enjoy the added variety of other strained juices available in several combination flavors.

The vitamin C content of all Gerber juices is standardized at a high level. All are strained for bottle-feeding to young babies. The doctor may suggest starting juice with a small amount, diluted with water. This is rapidly increased to at least 2 ounces of the full-strength juice. Older babies usually like a full can. Prior to weaning time, the tasty juices are ideal for practicing cup-feeding.

STARTING SOLIDS

Just as you follow the doctor's advice on your baby's formula and vitamin supplements, you will let him direct the addition of solid foods to baby's diet. He should decide when your baby is ready for them, suggest what should be served and schedule the order in which they should be added.

Doctors have varied opinions on when solids should be started. But there is widespread medical agreement that appropriate cereals and strained foods agree with babies almost from birth. On the other hand, there is seldom a reason why they need to be started so early, and it takes much time and patience to spoon-feed a newborn baby. That's why the majority of doctors delay the starting of cereals and/or strained food until sometime within the baby's second or third month. The family and baby have made many adjustments by this time, so solids can be introduced under more favorable circumstances.

The doctors who start babies on solids in the second and third months don't expect large quantities to be consumed. The main idea is to give baby plenty of time to get used to spoon-feeding before there is a great nutritional need for solid foods. Knowing this, you can offer the first solids in a relaxed frame of mind, without worrying about how well they are accepted the first day, the first week or even the first month.

Starting solid foods is a milestone in your baby's development. The "feel" of the spoon and of cereal or strained food will be puzzling. Movements of the tongue and throat muscles, beyond those used in sucking and swallowing liquids, will have to be learned. The occasion calls for careful staging so that the first experience with solids will be relaxed and pleasant.

TIMING IS IMPORTANT

Try giving baby his first solid food when he is in a pleasant frame of mind. Morning is usually a good time. It should be when he is reasonably hungry—but not necessarily at the beginning of the meal. Babies vary greatly in the times that they are most receptive to new foods. It may take a bit of experimenting on your part to learn what works best with your young one.

Prepare a small portion of the first solid food recommended by the doctor. This probably will be precooked cereal but it might be plain strained fruit, vegetables or meat. Follow package directions for mixing cereal with formula or milk. You may want to make it a little thinner for the first few feedings. Strained foods are the right consistency as they come from the jar. If warmed, the food should be tested for body temperature by putting a drop on your wrist.

A small, narrow, shallow-bowled spoon is best for early feeding. The preferred style might be described as a "long-handled, after-dinner coffee spoon."

When the big experiment with solid food is to be made, hold the baby in your lap in a comfortable position. This should be similar to that used in breast- or bottle-feeding, but more upright. This familiar position helps the baby anticipate food. Also, the food is less likely to "go down the wrong way." Relax and put on your best smile. Remember that it's unimportant whether the first try is successful or not.

Take a small amount of the new food on the tip of the spoon and place it well back on the baby's tongue. His head may be tipped back slightly at the same time. This offers the best chance for the food being swallowed. Some authorities suggest making the food more liquid and letting the baby suck it from the tip of the spoon. With some babies, this may work better. However, it doesn't teach a new skill and there's more chance of the food being pushed out when the baby's tongue encounters a new "feel."

Even with the best method of introduction, your baby may spit out the first few portions of solid food. It has nothing to do with whether he likes or dislikes it. He simply doesn't know what to do with it. Whatever happens, present a calm, unconcerned front. Offer another bite or so in the same casual manner, giving baby plenty of time to get used to the idea. Avoid antagonizing him by holding him too tightly or using force or pressure. Make every effort to maintain the pleasant atmosphere you want your baby always to associate with eating.

The flavors and textures of Gerber strained baby foods are designed to encourage acceptance. Usually a baby will accept a new food or merely appear indifferent to it. The latter simply calls for a little more time and patience. But occasionally there will be signs of determined resistance or serious objection. When this happens, calmly remove the food and make a fresh start the next day. If the same thing occurs then, it might be better to forget that food for several days, or even weeks, moving on to a different food. There are so many alternates available you'll have no trouble finding foods baby likes, even if he's a "picky" eater—and few babies are.

NO FOOD IS A "MUST"

It is reassuring to know that there is no one food which your baby must eat to be healthy. Babies can get their nutrients from many different foods. If they strongly dislike some food or one doesn't agree with them, there are any number of alternate choices within each of the "basic 4" food groups.

Cereals are the most frequently prescribed first solid

foods. Cereals prepared especially for babies are bland and palatable to a baby's taste. Being thoroughly precooked and low in crude fiber, they are easily digested. They have a creamy texture and consistency when stirred into milk, formula or other liquid.

Because milk does not supply babies with enough iron or thiamine, Gerber cereals are enriched with these nutrients. This was done at the suggestion and with the approval of doctors, who widely prescribe an early use of these special baby cereals, partly to satisfy appetite but especially as a source of iron and thiamine. The iron is added in a selected form that is proven to be efficiently utilized by babies and young children.

Other important B-complex vitamins, calcium and phosphorus also have been added to these starting cereals as further aids to your baby's well-being. Cereals are good sources of calories, and most supply moderate amounts of protein. The specially designed nutritive values of baby cereals warrant their use throughout infancy and the toddler period.

You will find these cereals just as convenient and economical as they are nourishing. They mix with liquids instantly, requiring no cooking or straining. The smallest portion can be prepared without waste of cereal, fuel or time.

In addition to directing when cereal or other solid food is started, your doctor may be quite specific about which one to give first. His directions should be followed closely. But if he lets you select the first solid, Rice Cereal is a good choice because it agrees well with almost all babies. This can be followed by Barley Cereal and Oatmeal (two other "one-grain" cereals) and later by Mixed Cereal and High Protein Cereal, which are mixtures.

As you mix the chosen first cereal, follow this time-proven method for faster creamy smoothness. Stir the cereal into the liquid—not vice versa.

Now you're ready. Settle baby comfortably in your arms, relax, smile—and try the first spoonful.

LITTLE MEAT EATERS

At one time, meats were almost the last foods included

in the baby's diet. Even then, the high nutritive values and digestibility of lean meats were recognized. It was simply too much trouble and often too expensive to prepare them in proper form at home. Those problems were eliminated when strained and junior meats became available twenty-five years ago. They offer babies the nutritional benefits of lean meat in a suitable, convenient and economical form. Today, many doctors suggest that strained meats be started at about the same early age as cereals. Some even prefer that meat be the first solid food. Check with your baby's doctor to see what his preference is.

Each savory variety of strained and junior meat is prepared from carefully selected and trimmed meats. Through special processing, the fat content is kept at a minimum, natural juices are retained and texture and consistency are just right for easy feeding.

Meats supply many nutrients important to babies and young children. Foremost are their complete, high-quality proteins, which are used in the growth and maintenance of every body cell. Proteins are also constituents of many body regulators.

Meats provide a variety of minerals. They are among the best sources of iron and phosphorus, which are important in all body tissues. Liver is especially high in iron. "Trace minerals," needed in tiny amounts but very important to many body functions, occur in wide variety in meats.

Meats also supply essential vitamins. All are excellent sources of niacin and supply some riboflavin, vitamin B_6, vitamin B_{12} and thiamine. Pork is especially high in thiamine, heart is a good source of riboflavin and liver is one of the richest sources of vitamin A.

The plain strained meats are the best starting meats. By using them, you quickly learn which individual meats agree with your baby. Also, while a baby's capacity for strained foods is small, plain meats provide more nourishment per spoonful. Later, for variety, part of a baby's meat intake may come from Gerber High Meat Dinners and smaller amounts may be had from vegetables and meat combination dinners.

Strained meats are more concentrated than the strained

vegetables and fruits. Therefore it is well to introduce them more gradually. At first, feed only one or two spoonfuls, perhaps diluting it a little. Over a few days, reduce the liquid until you are giving your baby straight meat. Once the baby is used to meat, you would expect to feed from one-third to one-half jar per day. Older babies, who have graduated to junior meats, usually like about one-half jar per day.

EGG YOLKS COME NEXT

Even before special baby foods were marketed, doctors recommended egg yolk for young babies as a supplementary source of iron. Later, when the iron-rich, precooked baby cereals and strained meats became available, most parents found them more convenient to serve than home-prepared egg yolk.

Then Gerber introduced strained egg yolks, which are convenient to feed baby. They are also sterile and have a moist, custardlike consistency and pleasant flavor that babies seem to relish. Medical tests have shown that commercially strained egg yolks agree with many babies better than home-prepared yolks.

In addition to iron, egg yolks are a good source of high-quality protein, vitamin A and riboflavin. They may be used instead of meat in noon or evening meals or served with cereal for breakfast. Egg Yolks and Ham is nutritionally similar to plain egg yolks and offers pleasant variety to older babies and toddlers.

There are approximately 3¼ yolks in a jar of strained egg yolks. Two tablespoonfuls equal one yolk. Appropriate servings range from one-third to one-half jar.

NOW VEGETABLES AND FRUITS

Your doctor will probably recommend beginning strained vegetables and fruits shortly after your baby is started on cereal and/or meat. This is likely to be within the baby's second or third month, the introduction of individual varieties being interspersed with the addition of new varieties of cereal and meat.

The chief contribution of vegetables and fruits is a variety of vitamins and minerals. However, individual items may vary greatly in which and how much of each nutrient they provide. In general, green and yellow vegetables and yellow fruits have high vitamin A values. Most fruits and vegetables contain some vitamin C but citrus fruits are the best contributors of this vitamin. Green vegetables supply appreciable iron. Used in wide variety, vegetables and fruits are among the best sources of trace minerals.

Serving your baby many kinds of vegetables and fruits helps build good food habits. These foods provide a wide variety of taste experiences at a time when food acceptances are most easily established. In later life, when parents no longer control the youngster's diet, such acceptances are difficult—sometimes impossible—to establish.

Back in 1933, when "baby foods" were new, Dr. Manuel Glazier of Boston reported on a study made on 231 babies to determine what happened when strained vegetables and fruits were fed as early as one month of age. Even these young babies digested the strained foods easily. Dr. Glazier concluded, "that the study showed the group fed solids early in infancy had better nutrition and better food and bowel habits and fewer food dislikes than the group fed solids in later infancy." Since then, his findings have been substantiated over and over.

It's a good idea to start with the plain strained vegetables and fruits before introducing those that are mixtures. And, as suggested before, each new product should be tried as the only new food three or four days before moving on to another.

Once a vegetable or fruit has been introduced and accepted, baby can be expected to eat one-third to one-half jar at a feeding. These are typical portions, but if your baby accepts less or wants more, why not respect his individuality?

Not less than two different servings of strained vegetables per day, at least one of them green or yellow, is a good dietary pattern. In addition, you will want to include at least one, but probably more, strained fruits per day. A word of caution: perhaps you'll discover, as many parents have, that your baby accepts fruits more readily than vegetables. Be careful not to let this result in an overuse of fruits to the exclusion of vegetables, which generally have higher nutritive values. In such cases, it might be better to serve the vegetables first, while the baby is hungry, and withhold the fruit until later, for dessert.

VEGETABLES AND MEAT COMBINATIONS

After your baby is accustomed to the many varieties of plain vegetables, plain meats and cereals, you can provide new taste experiences through serving strained combinations. These pleasantly combine vegetables, cereals and meat. Baby's first-year acquaintance with mixed flavors is an important step in his learning to accept grown-up foods later on. quite similar to the plain vegetables. Their proper use in a baby's menu is as alternates for vegetables. In other words, quite similar to the plain vegetables. In other words, they would be only part of a meal that would also contain plain meats, egg yolks, cottage cheese, or other high-protein food.

These vegetables and meat combinations have a just-right consistency for babies. Serve about the same size portions as vegetables—one-third to one-half jar.

HIGH MEAT DINNERS

The high meat dinners, first developed and introduced by Gerber, are combinations of a substantial amount (30 percent) of meat plus vegetables and cereal. Served in generous portions, they make tasty main courses that offer about the same nutritive values as meals made up of smaller portions of plain meats, plain vegetables and cereal.

As with other combinations, the high meat dinners should be introduced after the baby has become accustomed to the many plain foods available. Once started and accepted, they should be alternated with meals of plain foods to give widest variety and interest. When high meat dinners are used as the entire main course, a whole jar would be the usual serving.

It's natural for you to wonder how the high meat dinners, the vegetable and meat combinations and the plain strained and junior meats compare in protein content. Gerber High Meat Dinners contain about 8 grams of protein per

4½-ounce jar. Gerber strained and junior meats average about 19 grams of protein per 4½ ounces (1¼ jar). Gerber strained and junior vegetables and meat combinations, about 2.8 grams protein per 4½ ounces.

Cottage Cheese with Pineapple (green label) was developed by Gerber. It is low in fat and has a protein content similar to that of High Meat Dinners. Like them, it is intended for use as a main dish. Cottage cheese is also a good source of calcium and riboflavin. The pleasant blend of flavors is readily accepted by babies. Serve at room temperature.

HOW BIG IS BABY

Many young mothers tell us that their babies have learned to drink from a glass or a cup very early. It's a very good idea to accustom the little one to drinking from something other than the bottle—then, when weaning time comes, you're likely to have much less difficulty. Give water or orange juice from a cup or glass, starting at three or four months. Don't push—if baby doesn't like the idea, give up for the moment and come back to it a bit later. And don't expect him to be neat—the first few tries will result in most of the liquid spilling down his front. But you'll have put a good bib with a catch-all pocket on him, so it won't matter. You'll be surprised at how quickly he'll get the hang of drinking from cup or glass.

Time will hurry by, and all at once your baby will be six months old. By this time he will be eating a wide variety —and, probably, relishing every mouthful because he's growing rapidly.

He'll be eating cereal, egg yolk, several kinds of meats, a number of different fruits and vegetables, cottage cheese. How will you plan his menu for the day? That's up to you. Baby doesn't know that most adults eat eggs or cereal for breakfast, a reasonably light lunch, their main meal at dinner time, so put him on any schedule that suits the convenience of both of you. One division of baby foods through the day that seems to work well, young mothers tell us, is cereal and egg yolk at breakfast, juice at midmorning, vegetable and meat for lunch, high meat dinner and fruit at dinner time. But there are no rules—let your convenience and what works best for your baby be your guides.

POTATOES AND PASTAS

Strained sweet potatoes can be fed as soon as any of the other plain vegetables. In fact, their pleasant flavor and high vitamin A and iron values have made them popular as one of the earliest strained foods.

Babies over six months of age often receive a taste or two of baked or mashed white potato. The small portions don't contribute much nutritionally, but it's well for babies to learn to like a food so widely used in family meals. Most of the strained and junior "dinners" contain some white potato, so this is another means through which baby can become acquainted with this family food.

Many families use macaroni, spaghetti, noodles and other pastas extensively. It's well for older babies in these families to have a chance to learn to like them. Enriched macaroni and spaghetti and egg noodles are included in a number of junior foods, combined with other wholesome ingredients and suitably seasoned for babies.

BAKED GOODS

When your baby starts teething, hard breads may be offered in limited amounts. They're something on which the baby might bite and are a first step in self-feeding. Teething biscuits, zwieback, and finger-shaped pieces of dry toast or bread are favored first-year breads.

Gerber Teething Biscuits are especially shaped for easy grasping and are hard-baked for biting satisfaction and for preventing crumbling—a safety feature, since it's easy for crumbs to go down a baby's throat "the wrong way." That's also a good reason why babies shouldn't eat breads or other dry foods while lying down.

Usually babies don't get much nutritive benefit from breads because they actually eat only a small part of each piece. They do more biting and sucking than chewing and swallowing. But toddlers generally consume the full portion. From this age on, baked goods should be chosen for nutritive value as well as physical properties.

Gerber Cookies are made from a variety of wholesome ingredients. They have twice the average protein content of ordinary cookies and are thinly glazed with an icing containing important B vitamins. They were developed with the high nutritional needs of toddlers and preschool children in mind.

If given a free hand, most babies and young children would eat teething biscuits and cookies in excessive quantity to the exclusion of other important foods. You be the judge of the proper quantity—once again, you're the one in control, not baby. One or two teething biscuits or four or five cookies per day are plenty. They should be given as part of a meal or as a suitably timed snack between meals. Their continuous use, as a "pacifier," is unwise.

"I WANT TO DO IT MYSELF"

The point of baby's wanting to help spoon-feed himself will probably come quite early. He will greatly enjoy holding a spoon and trying to find his mouth with it while you feed him with another spoon. He can best manage a short-handled, large-bowled spoon. When the baby begins drinking his milk from a cup, you can reduce spilling if the cup contains only a small amount. Then you can increase the amount as the baby becomes more adept at managing the cup.

You'll want to start slowly. A sip or two at a time is enough in the beginning. But at bedtime, or when the baby is tired, don't insist upon his drinking from a cup. Let him have the comfort of the familiar bottle.

THE MILK REBELLION

Often, when babies are around a year old, they rebel at drinking milk. If yours does, there's no need to worry. You can use extra milk in his food or dress it up as a fruit shake or serve it as a custard. A young mother tells us she's found that her babies forget all about the milk rebellion when she serves the milk in a brightly colored cup (plastic, so that it doesn't break if dropped).

Even the best baby will rebel occasionally, sometimes against food, sometimes against other things. Relax; there's no need to force the issue. Showing a mind of his own indicates that baby is growing up. This applies to wanting to feed himself, too. So encourage it, no matter what a mess he makes at first. A good bib protects his clothes. Plastic or newspaper protects the floor. Like everything else in life, practice makes perfect!

You will find that it is always best to stay calm and confident (or, at least, to *appear* that way). If *you* believe you know what is best for your child, *he* will absorb that belief. A small child cannot know what is best for him and needs loving guidance and gentle but firm discipline. The child who is never corrected and is allowed to do as he pleases grows up feeling that his parents don't care enough about him to bother.

WHEN APPETITE LAGS

There are times, of course, when teething or illness causes lagging appetite. Then, naturally, you'll want to do what you can to make mealtimes more interesting. Sometimes the baby will reject new foods; in that case, stay with proven favorites until he is feeling bouncy again. At other times, you may want to use new foods or food combinations to tempt his lagging appetite.

Mealtime dawdling and saying no to everything are common problems during the toddler phase, and we get many anxious letters from mothers about that problem. This is another time to remain calm or at least to maintain an outward show of calm. You will find that ignoring the problem will end it much more quickly than becoming upset and attempting to coax or force a child to eat. But you might give a little thought to *why* he is acting this way.

Have you been serving oversized portions? Foods he doesn't like? Singing songs or making funny faces to coax him to eat, so that he prolongs the meal in order to see the entire show? When the answers are all no and he is obviously stalling to get attention at any price, a good solution is to remove the food after a sensible length of time—and no between-meal snacks! It isn't all that long until the next meal, and he won't be harmed by going a bit hungry for a little while. You'll find such a course of action will do wonders for his appetite. Dawdling and saying no are much less fun for him this way.

Here are a few tips on making mealtimes more pleasant for *you,* too. When your baby is starting to feed himself and gets more food on the outside than the inside, you might want to spread a sizable piece of plastic or several newspapers on the floor under the high chair. After the meal you can wipe the plastic clean or dispose of the newspapers, which is so much easier than cleaning the floor.

You might try serving fruits, desserts and juices to the toddler in paper cups. They won't break if he drops them, and they can be thrown away after use. This cuts down on the dishwashing. The gay designs and bright colors of these cups make them appealing to youngsters, too. And, in nice weather, what about taking your toddler outdoors for a picnic meal? Children love that, even if you go no farther than your own backyard. It will be fun for you, too.

IT'S TIME FOR DESSERT

During the first year, it's wise to emphasize fruits as your baby's dessert. They are neither overly sweet nor unduly high in calories in relation to other nutrients.

Next to fruits, custards, puddings and rennet-custards, containing milk and only moderately sweetened, are preferred. The wholesome Gerber desserts are based on milk, eggs or fruits and are lightly sweetened. Needless to say, more concentrated sweets—high in calories and low in general nutritive value—cannot be recommended for infants and preschool children.

Babies and children don't have to learn to like sweets as they do other foods. They accept them instinctively. That's another reason why there's no advantage in introducing them as early as other foods. More than with any other food, the use of desserts should be individualized. They are appropriate "extras" for large active babies with appetites and calorie needs beyond those met by reasonable amounts of milk, meats, vegetables, fruits and cereals. Some small babies with poor appetites and food acceptances are probably better off without desserts. Let your doctor direct you on your baby's use of desserts.

GROWING UP

It's generally agreed that keeping babies on only liquids and strained foods beyond the first year is an invitation to later feeding problems. Most doctors recommend a gradual shift from strained to junior foods when babies are eight to ten months old. The "minced" texture of Gerber junior foods is safe at even earlier ages if your doctor thinks your baby is ready for coarser foods.

Start the switch with softer junior foods like the fruits. Then move on to the firmer junior vegetables, "dinners" and meats. Most of the baby's favorite strained foods are available in the junior texture, and it is well to begin with these. Later, add the increasing variety of "casserole" type junior foods which cater to the "growing-up" tastes of toddlers.

As a final step in the transition to family foods, serve "finger foods," such as meat sticks and the new Toddler Meals. These are interesting and hearty "main course" casseroles. A six-ounce jar, with milk and a fruit or dessert, is an ample meal.

Many parents wonder about serving cereals during the junior-food age. While no longer necessary from the standpoint of texture, the precooked baby cereals offer several nutritional advantages because of their generous fortification with iron and B vitamins. During the toddler years, when a smaller volume of food is eaten, these higher nutritive values can be especially important. Gerber High Protein Cereal is both nutritious and appealing for toddlers and preschoolers.

You have the final responsibility for protecting baby-food quality. This continues from the time it leaves the grocery shelf until the baby has eaten the last portion.

For over ten years, Gerber has used special caps to guide mothers. Before opening, the small circle at the center of the cap should be concave (sink downward). If something has caused loss of vacuum, the circle on the cap will be convex (curve upward). When buying or starting to open jars of Gerber food, check for the concave (downward) circle. Then, for further assurance, listen for the "pop" when first opening the jar at home to feed the baby.

After opening, baby foods should be out of the refrigerator only long enough to remove each serving. The jars hold only two or three portions, and the juice cans, but one or two. This permits full use of the contents within a safe period, if properly handled.

At feeding time, transfer just the portion to be fed to the serving dish. If served warm, heat by placing the dish in simmering water or warming dish. *When only part of a jar's contents will be fed, it is better not to heat the food in the jar or to feed directly from it.* The increased contamination and delay in chilling can cause more rapid spoilage. Repeated heating also lessens palatability and can lower nutritive values. *Saliva from the baby's spoon may liquefy foods by "digesting" them.*

It is more convenient and sanitary to refrigerate unserved baby foods in the original jar or can. During processing, their inside surfaces have been sterilized, along with the food. Transferring to another container offers more opportunity for contamination and faster spoilage. The U.S. Department of Agriculture endorses refrigerating saveovers in the original jar or can.

For best protection of quality, keep jars and cans covered during refrigeration. This reduces contamination with airborne bacteria, yeasts and molds, which cause spoilage. It also keeps food from drying and may prevent loss of certain nutrients. Jars are easily reclosed with their twist-type caps. Cans may be covered with aluminum foil, plastic film or waxed paper.

Packages of baby cereal should be stored in a cool, dry place. Keep them apart from soaps, cleaners, drugs and strongly flavored vegetables to prevent the absorption of foreign odors. Baby cereals should also be isolated from other grain products that might be a source of insect infestation.

IF FEEDING PROBLEMS DEVELOP

Preventing feeding problems is much easier than correcting them. But if, in spite of your good intentions, feeding problems do develop, try to determine the causes. Then decide on—and firmly adhere to—a course of action.

What is a feeding problem? It occurs when a child fails to eat as his parents expect him to. Whether these expectations are right or wrong, the result is the same—tensions which create an unhappy family situation.

Most feeding problems fall into one of two classes. One is the child's not eating enough, or what the parents think is "enough." The other is the child's not eating specific foods the parents would like accepted. Usually these are "good-for-you" foods, such as milk, meat and vegetables. It's well for these parents to remember that a child's appetite is a good guide to how much he should eat and that there is no one food which a child must eat.

Few feeding problems develop in the first year. Growth is rapid, food needs are high and babies' appetites are good. You'll probably be satisfied with the amount baby eats during that time. It's in the second and third years, when growth rate, food needs and intake diminish, that trouble is more likely to occur.

Everybody likes attention. A toddler is likely to get it the first few times he eats less than usual. Whether your reaction takes the form of mild coaxing or forced feeding, the child knows he's being noticed. Pretty soon he knows that refusing food is an attention-getter. It can be even more fun than eating. The remedy is to be alert to and ignore the lowered intake. Most toddlers go through a normal stage of saying no to everything, even when they don't mean it. If it happens to attract attention, saying no at mealtime can get to be quite a game and a habit. It should be ignored like any other play for attention.

Some youngsters use refusal of food as a bargaining device in obtaining certain desires. It's most unwise ever to bribe a child to eat. Families should always maintain the attitude that eating is a privilege, not a favor.

Babies are great imitators and quickly follow the example of a parent or older brother or sister. When they eat at the family table, family members can help by being willing to set good examples. Only favorable attitudes, by word or gesture, should be expressed toward food. Too much discussion, even of the favorable type, is unwise.

Mealtime surroundings should be clean, bright and cheerful, and the atmosphere, a happy one. There should be no unnecessary distractions which draw a child's attention from eating. Decorations, conversation or activity should not be overdone. A desire to play can be a strong distraction for a toddler. Sometimes firm policies have to be made.

Wise parents use every opportunity to develop and maintain a toddler's interest in food. Even though it's slow and untidy, self-feeding should be encouraged. Protect the floor and put the baby on his own. The food may often miss its target but baby's interest will be maintained through his sense of accomplishment. Toward the end of the meal, when the baby tires, he'll usually appreciate help with the last few spoonfuls.

Mealtime discipline, such as stress on table manners, can deter a toddler's interest in food. Training of this type is more effective in the later preschool period when there's better muscular coordination. In the meantime, some progress might be made through imitation of good examples set by older family members.

Dawdling at mealtime is a common problem. Like refusal of food, it can easily become an attention-getter and is therefore better ignored. Allowance should be made for a small child's lack of skill. But if a meal stretches beyond a reasonable period, it's well to remove the food calmly and without comment.

Most feeding problems appear to be psychological in origin and nature. Occasionally the blame may rest in the diet itself. Diets too high in fat, sweets or starch or too low in certain vitamins might inhibit appetite. The spacing of meals also affects food acceptance. When appetite is poor, the interval between meals might be increased. Sometimes feeding smaller portions helps.

Sufficient fresh air, exercise and sleep are other factors known to have a favorable influence on appetite. In today's casual living, most youngsters get enough of these—but they are worth checking if appetite is poor.

If you are truly concerned over your baby's appetite and/or eating habits, talk the problem over with your doctor and follow his suggestions. If he says "don't worry"—don't!

5

Each Day, Every Day

Almost as soon as you bring your baby home from the hospital, the washing begins—bathing the baby and laundering his clothing, diapers, bed linen, blankets. You'll soon find that bath time is fun, both for you and for the baby, when approached in the right spirit. Similarly, it's a positive pleasure to see soiled items become fresh, fragrant and like new once more.

Take advantage of all modern conveniences within your means—for instance, automatic washers and dryers, diaper services, disposable diapers, to name just a few of the modern wonders that simplify your job. At the same time, you retain the instinctive knowledge of how to handle and care for this precious infant of yours.

Relax and take things easy at first. You can keep baby clean and comfortable with sponge baths until after the navel and circumcision are healed. Then, when you're stronger —and more sure of yourself, less timid about handling the baby—and when you've more or less established a daily routine, you can have a regular time for bathing baby—a time you'll both look forward to.

SPONGE BATHS

A table—or other flat surface—or your lap, as you choose, may be used for giving baby a sponge bath. (An apron will keep your clothes dry, a plastic apron will waterproof you. If you use a plastic apron, you'll want something between it and the baby, such as a diaper or a soft bath towel, both to absorb water and to keep soapy baby from slipping.) If you put the baby on a tabletop or a similar surface, you'll want waterproof material under him to protect the tabletop and something warmer over it—again, a towel or a diaper. If you're using a hard surface, more will be needed—padding of some sort, a folded blanket or quilt.

Wash baby's face and scalp with a washcloth rung out in clear, warm water. Once or twice a week, soap his scalp, being careful not to let any soap run down into his eyes, then rinse well. Wash the rest of his body with a soaped washcloth or with your soapy hand—sometimes it's easier to soap your right hand while you hold baby securely on your lap with your left hand. Then rinse with the washcloth rinsed and wrung out in clear water—two rinses, to make sure of getting rid of all the soap. Pay attention to all the creases, both when you're washing and when you're rinsing.

A "REAL" BATH

Many doctors suggest bathing the baby just before the 10 A.M. feeding, but generally they make this suggestion because they feel this may be the most convenient time for you. If it's not, almost any other time will do. Usually right after a feeding is not a good bathing time because you'll want baby to nap then—maybe you'll want to rest, as well—and bathing makes most babies wakeful. (Some it soothes to sleep, however.) Choose a time that suits your schedule. Often just before the 6 P.M. feeding is the chosen time so that Daddy, too, can share the pleasure of seeing baby in the bathtub or even take over his bathing.

What do you bathe baby in? Almost anything that will

hold water has been used as a baby bath. Perhaps you've bought or have been given a bathinette. Or use a dishpan, a small enamelware or plastic tub, the kitchen sink, the bathroom washbasin, whatever is most convenient for you. Baby couldn't care less. (Not the big bathtub, though—it's too hard on your back and knees.) Stand during the bath or sit on a stool—perhaps the latter if most of your day seems to be spent on your feet.

Before you bring baby to the bath, make sure you're ready for him. Assemble everything you need—towel, washcloth, soap (any good baby soap is fine), absorbent cotton to clean his ears and nose if necessary, powder or lotion if you use them, clean diaper and pins and whatever else you're going to put on him after the bath. And an apron for you—again, plastic will keep you dry. If you're bathing him in a bathinette away from a faucet, don't forget water to fill the tub.

How warm should the water be? Between 90 and 100 degrees. You can use a bath thermometer if you like, but it's not necessary. The water should feel just comfortably warm to your elbow. At first, until you get the knack of holding baby with one hand while you wash him with the other, use a very small amount of water. The room should be warm enough so that his wet body won't feel chilled. Pad the bottom of the tub—this is usually not necessary if you use a bathinette—with a towel or a diaper. If you are bathing baby in the sink or washbasin, turn off the hot tap before turning off the cold—otherwise the tap may stay hot and baby may touch it with a waving fist. This is an especially wise precaution when baby is old enough to thrash about considerably.

Now get the baby.

Lower him gently into the water, your left arm (unless you are left-handed) behind him so that your hand is under his left armpit, your wrist and lower arm supporting his neck and head. Wash his face first, with a wrung-out washcloth, using water only—no soap. Shampoo only twice a week, soaping first, then rinsing twice with a damp washcloth. (Hint from a young friend of mine: a tiny dab of cold cream above the eyebrows sidetracks suds and avoids the sting of soap in little eyes. There are also nonsting baby shampoos available if you fear you'll inadvertently get soap in baby's eyes.)

Next, soap baby all over, paying particular attention to creases and the diaper area. Do this with a soaped washcloth or your soaped hand—again, you may find the soaped hand easier, because your other hand will be occupied holding the baby. Rinse twice with a wrung-out washcloth, making sure that you remove all soap. Soap gently—he's really not very dirty, although a few years from now you'll wonder if you can ever get him clean short of using a scrub brush! But for now, remember how tender that brand-new skin is! Remember, too, that a soaped baby is a slippery baby. Be sure you have a good grip on him.

FUN TIME FOR BABY

Bath time can be fun time, particularly when your young one is old enough to sit up and play a little in the tub. There's something endlessly fascinating to babies in slapping their hands flat on the water for an apparently very satisfying sound-and-splash result. Bath toys—a duck, a boat, anything suitable for play in the water—delight babies a little older. But a baby of almost any age will find your delight in bathing him "catching." Make bath time a fun time, a relaxed time, and baths will become so enjoyable that you can use them for easing your baby out of a cranky mood.

SPECIAL PROBLEMS, SPECIAL CARE

You need only wash the outer part of the ear—don't try to probe into the canal. The wax formed there is for a purpose—to protect the inner ear and clean it.

Eyes need no special care. They are constantly being bathed by tears, not only when baby is crying but all the time, and tears are much better for the young one's eyes than anything you could put into them. Healthy eyes need no eyedrops or other treatment.

The mouth, too, requires no help from you to keep it clean. Later on there'll be teeth and your toddler will learn to brush them, but until then don't make any attempt to clean his mouth. It's fine the way nature made it.

Fingernails do need care—they must be cut so that the baby doesn't scratch himself and others. Many mothers make this job part of the bath-time routine, but when the baby is asleep is actually a better time, a number of young mothers suggest, particularly if your young one is a fist clencher. Or catch him when he's very drowsy. There are special manicure scissors with little balls where ordinary scissors have points just made for this task. Or use a small pair of ordinary scissors or clippers—many mothers find that clippers are easier to handle. Another young mother suggests holding the baby in your lap in front of a mirror and giving him that "manicure" while he's absorbed in watching his reflection.

Especially in winter, when the heat is on and dries the air, dried mucus collects in the baby's nose. In most cases the nose itself solves the problem. Hairs in the lining of the nose push the mucus forward, collecting as it goes any dust or dirt that may have gotten in. This mucus gathers on the larger hairs at the openings of the nostrils. This causes a tickling sensation and the baby sneezes or rubs the accumulation out. If necessary, or if the baby seems to have trouble breathing in a warm, dry room, moisten a corner of a washcloth or a piece of cotton twisted to a point and gently remove the dried mucus. Older children breathe through their mouths when their noses are stuffed up, but babies don't seem to be able to.

If your baby gets a little rash—many babies do, at one time or another—a couple of tablespoonfuls of baking soda in the bath water helps soothe the irritation. Baby powder helps to foil prickly heat; so does brushing the baby's hair upward at the back of his neck. Of course, if he has a rash that persists, you'll want to ask your doctor about it.

GOOD THINGS COME TO AN END

The bath is over, and baby has to come out of the tub. When he's very young, you simply lift him out and that's that. When he gets older, you may have some difficulty getting him out of the tub because he enjoys his bath so much. (One young mother wrote me that she lets the water out—that spoils the fun and baby is willing to be taken out of the tub.)

Dry baby carefully, patting and blotting rather than

rubbing. Pay special attention to the creases, for moisture left there can cause irritation. When he's thoroughly dry, smooth on powder or baby lotion. If you use powder, don't sprinkle him directly with it—powder your hand, turning away so that there won't be a cloud of powder for baby to inhale. Then apply the powder from your hand to the baby.

SOME BATH-TIME IDEAS

If you bathe your baby in a rubber-lined folding bathinette, you'll find that using a water conditioner will keep the lining soft as well as clean. The conditioner prevents soap curd from remaining behind to stiffen the lining. Incidentally, this works well with baby's waterproof pants, too—remember that at laundry time!

Plastic or plastic-coated wallpaper on the wall behind the baby's bath area allows you and baby to splash and enjoy yourselves at bath time without worrying about possible stains on the wall. Another bath-area idea: an inexpensive spice rack is great for holding lotion, powder, swabs, cotton, pins and so on.

A young mother in Hawaii tells me that she finds a waterproof surfer's watch a great help. It's rugged, inexpensive and there's no need to remove it while bathing the baby or doing the laundry. Wearing it, she always knows the time and can save her good watch for dress-up occasions.

EVERY DAY IS WASH DAY

Keeping baby clean is only half the battle—you must keep his clothes clean, too, and his bedclothes and towels and washcloths. The laundry does indeed begin to accumulate the moment you're home from the hospital.

Diapers! Perhaps you'll decide that the convenience of a diaper service is worth the cost. Perhaps you are on a tight budget and decide you had better launder diapers yourself. The diaper services do provide the diapers and a covered hamper that is deodorized and drip-proof. All you have to do is remove stools from diapers, to minimize the odor, before putting them in the hamper.

Disposable diaper liners will reduce the messiness of changing baby and doing the laundry. They also cut down on staining and aid in preventing diaper rash since they are treated with antibacterial agents.

If, like so many young mothers, you must watch every penny and would rather use that money for something other than diaper service or even disposable liners, you'll find that there's nothing difficult about washing diapers. The diapers are very important to your child's comfort, so you'll want to get them thoroughly clean, with no hard-water film making them stiff, nonabsorbent and irritating to baby's tender skin.

To start with, it's wise to rinse soiled diapers in the toilet to remove particles. Then soak them, along with the wet diapers, in a covered pail until you have enough to make a washer load.

When you have a load accumulated (and it *is* best to wash diapers separately from other laundry except that you might wash them with baby's wet sheets and sleepers), use the cotton or regular setting on the washer. Use the hottest water possible and your regular laundry compound. You'll want to use an extra rinse, if available, and if you use a fabric softener in the final rinse, pinning will be easier—though to maintain peak absorbency, you should omit the softener about every fourth laundering. Then dry completely in the dryer's normal cycle. There! Nothing difficult about that. And what a feeling of accomplishment it can give you, having things clean and fresh again with a minimum of work and expense!

The rest of your baby's clothing can be laundered with family garments of similar colors and fabrics—white clothes together, colored garments, cottons and so on. For all their tiny size and delicate appearance, baby's pretty outfits are quite practical and washable. Just follow a few basic tips, and you can easily retain the fresh colors and cozy texture of brand-new baby clothes.

GENTLE CARE FOR DELICATE FABRICS

Most knitted items can be washed in machines which have special cycles for delicate fabrics. Just remember to wash woolens in cool to lukewarm water and handle them as little as possible while wet. Sweaters hold their shape better if buttoned before washing. When hand-washing, press the garments

Dressing a wriggling baby—all babies wriggle—is a knack you will quickly get the hang of. *See page 11 for baby clothing tips.*

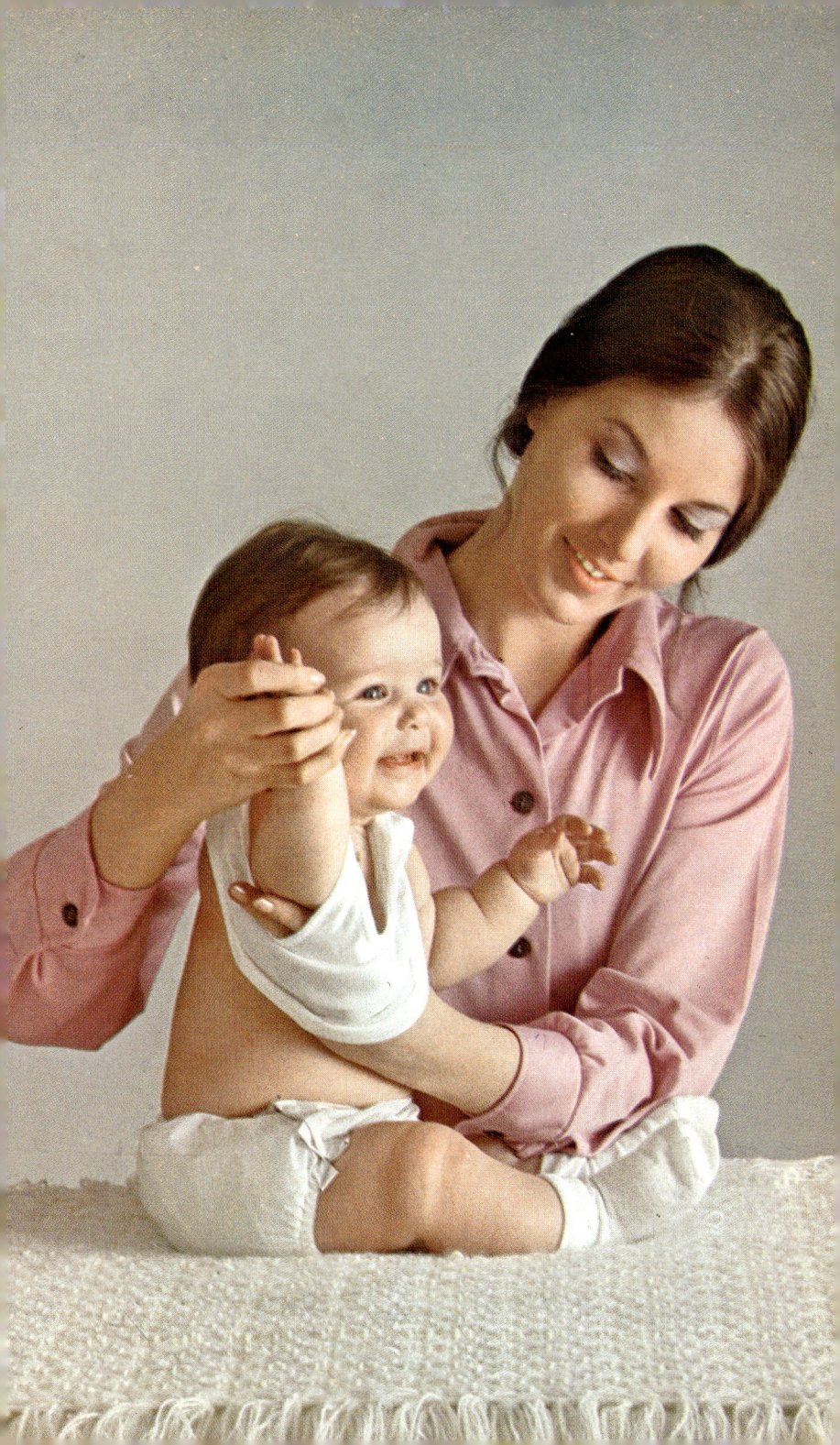

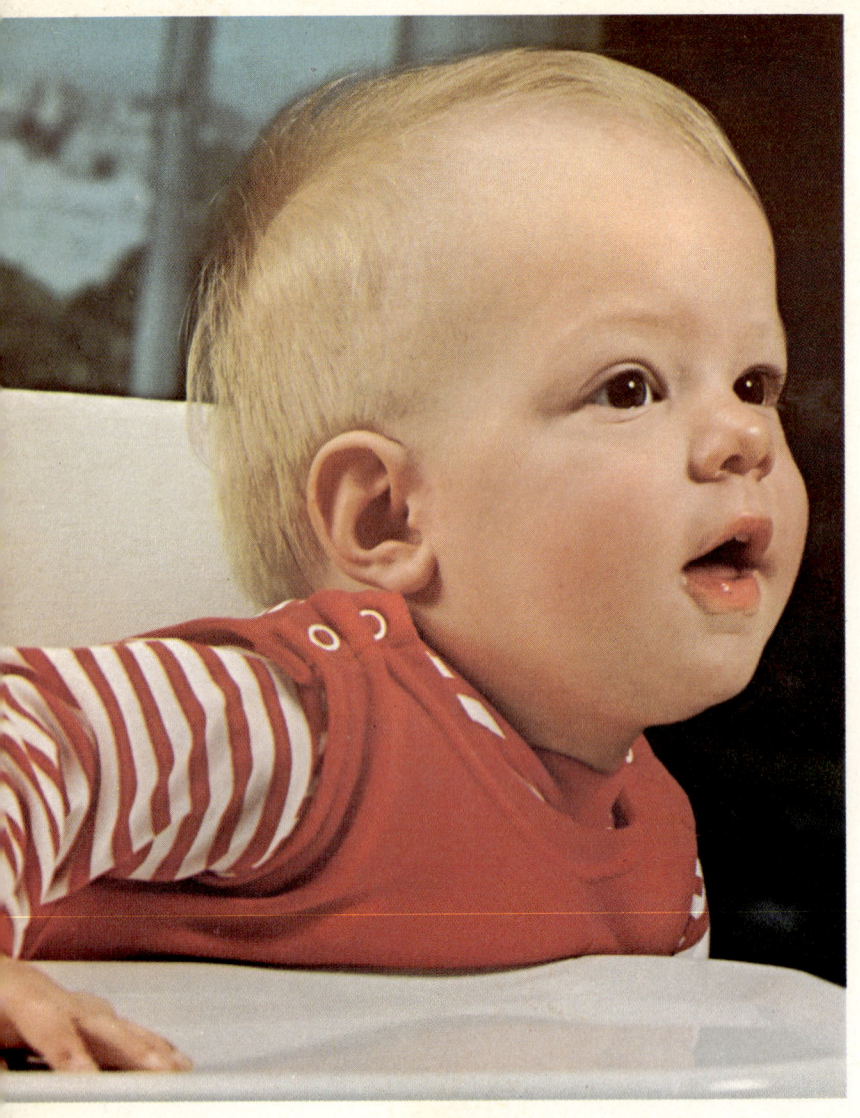

Bright colors catch baby's eye, clothes that fasten with grippers make dressing him easy. *See pages 13–14 for baby clothing tips.*

Cuddly sleepers keep baby cozy through the night and at naptime, even if he kicks off the covers. *See pages 69–71 for sleeping tips.*

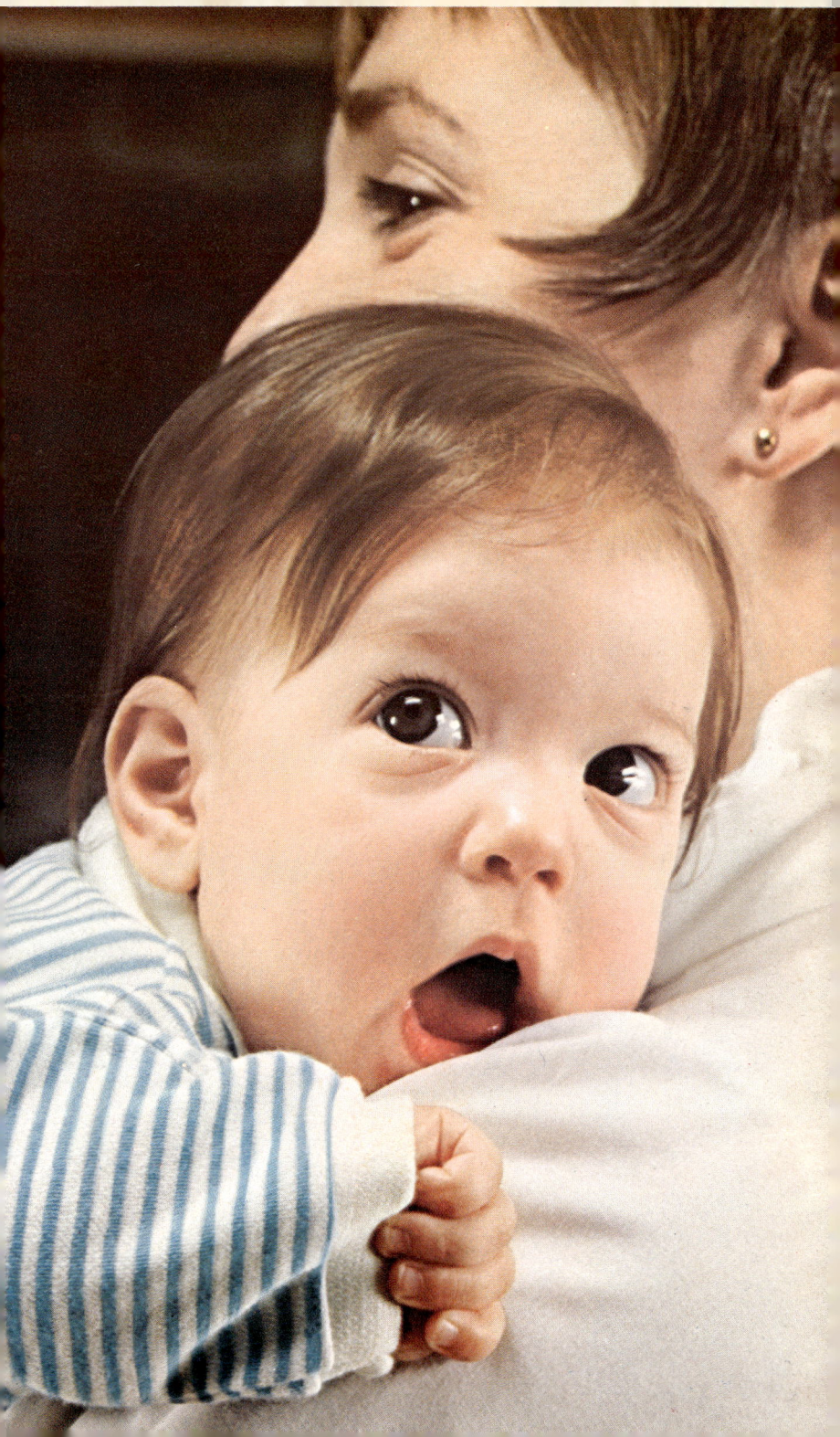

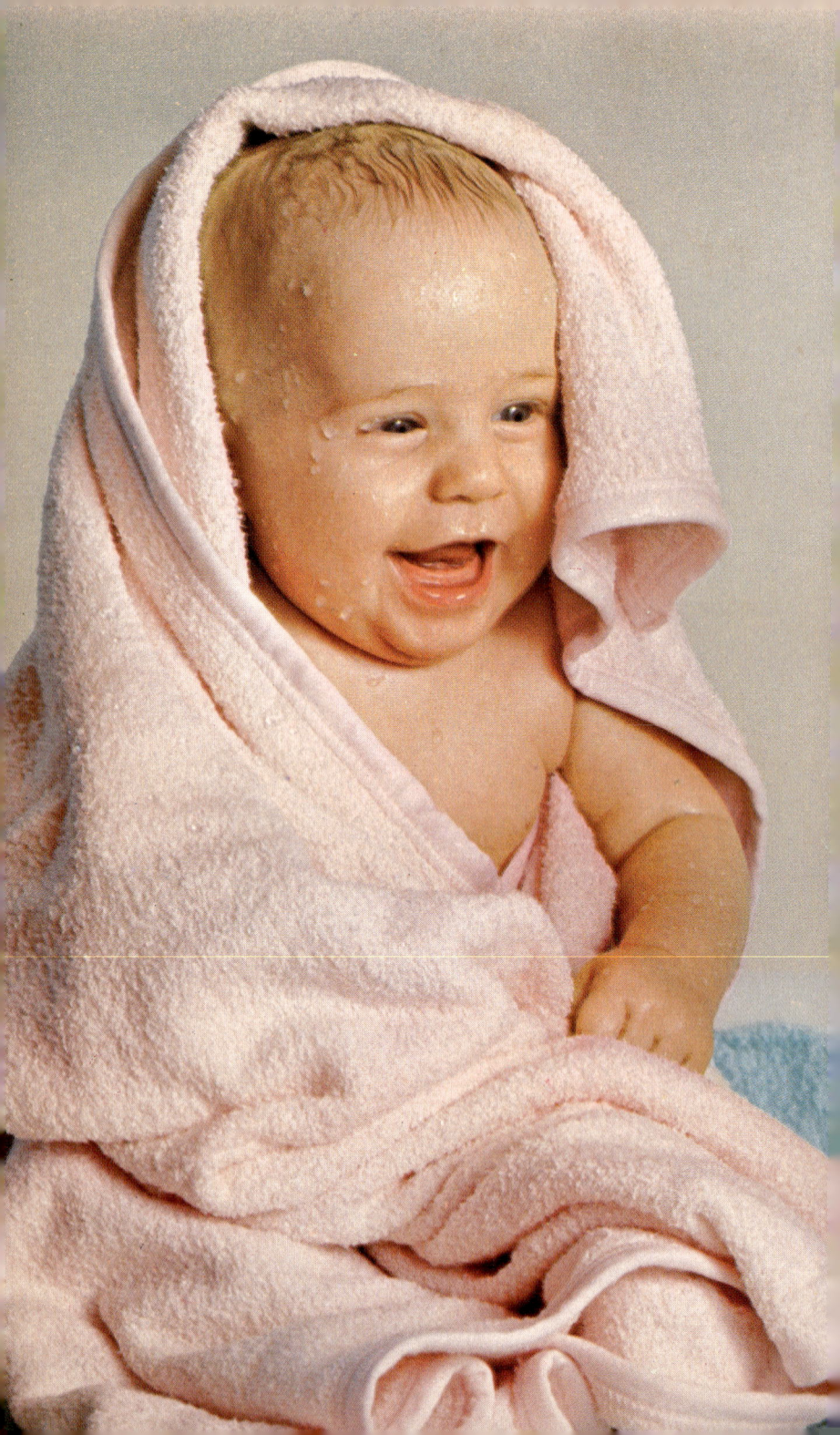

up and down gently through the suds—don't rub and twist them. Rinse, then wrap them in a thick bath towel to blot out the water. Block them to shape, and dry flat. Bonnets retain their shape better if stuffed with tissue paper.

Any stains should be pretreated, as many are set by hot water. You'll find it a good idea to mend any rips or tears before putting garments into the washer, for they can grow worse during laundering.

Waterproof plastic pants are best laundered in a mesh bag so that they won't "melt" to the side of the dryer's drum. Or you may prefer to hand-wash them with detergent and to air-dry them. Some soaps and bleaches decompose the plastic, making it stiff and brittle. We've found that detergents keep plastic pants soft and waterproof longer.

Baby's clothes aren't the only things that increase the laundry load. You'll find yourself washing more towels, aprons, sheets, bath rugs—and presently, when the baby's a little older, slipcovers, bedspreads and throw rugs, too. Water conditioners help to get them extra clean, removing old washing film, and make them smell deliciously fresh.

There'll be toys to wash, too. Babies do love soft, huggable stuffed toys. In buying them, it's wise to make sure they're washable, or you may find that the toy most essential to baby's happiness is growing steadily more disreputable while washing would destroy it. Most stuffed toys can be machine-laundered or washed with a soft brush and soap suds.

While we're on the subject, do make certain that the toy's eyes, nose and mouth, if not part of the toy itself, are securely fastened on. Such things can find their way into baby's mouth or nose or ears.

Make up your mind never to throw away a cherished old toy and substitute for it one that seems to you more desirable because it's clean and new or because someone dear to you— the baby's grandmother, perhaps—has sent it as a gift. Usually a baby chooses one toy that he is particularly fond of. Nobody knows why this particular choice—to you it may seem the least attractive toy he has. Never mind—it's his, and it's very dear to him. No matter how shabby it gets, let him have it. If it falls apart, mend it for him. He doesn't care what it looks like—to him it is beautiful and his own,

Most babies consider bath time one of the highlights of the day. A large soft towel makes drying quick and easy. *See pages 59–63.*

and to deprive him of it is unkind and entirely unnecessary.

WHAT IS THE RIGHT TEMPERATURE?

Mothers worry a lot—unnecessarily, most doctors believe—about whether the temperature is right in the room where the baby sleeps, whether he has enough covers to keep him warm. If mothers make mistakes about temperature, experts say, it's usually on the side of keeping baby too warm, not too cold.

Newborns who weigh under five pounds, as you probably know, are kept in incubators. That's because the mechanisms for keeping their bodies at a comfortable, safe temperature do not work well at this weight.

However, when the baby weighs over five pounds, his body can regulate its own heat in a room that is neither very hot nor very cold—one that has a temperature of, say, between sixty-eight and seventy-two degrees. By the time he has reached eight pounds, his "thermostat" is working well, and he can regulate his own body temperature within reasonable bounds. Besides, by now he's building up a layer of fat that serves as insulation to help him keep warm. In cool weather his sleeping-room temperature can drop to sixty degrees and he'll keep warm, provided that he is covered or wrapped in a sleeping bag. You, too, would require covers in a sixty-degree room.

In fact, by the time your baby weighs eight pounds or more, you can be the judge of whether he is too hot, too cold or just comfortable by the way you, yourself, react to the temperature of the room. He'll react about the same way unless, of course, he wears many more or fewer clothes than you do. If you find the room chilly enough to put on a sweater, you might put one on baby, too. When the room warms up and you take yours off, remove his as well. It's that simple. A room whose temperature is between sixty-eight and seventy-two degrees is usually quite comfortable for all—babies, children and adults.

HOW MUCH CLOTHING IS THE RIGHT AMOUNT?

Your baby is more likely to be too warmly dressed than not warmly enough—that's because you worry about him and want to make sure he's comfortable and doesn't get chilled. Many babies are well-rounded, and generally they need a little less clothing than an adult does—and usually quite a lot less than an adult *thinks* they need. Being overdressed isn't good for baby. If he's always too warmly dressed, his body's ability to adjust to the temperature around him will be lowered.

Don't try to judge whether or not baby is warm enough by feeling his hands. A baby's hands generally feel cool even when he's plenty warm enough. Instead, feel his arms or his legs or his neck—those are all better indicators of whether or not he is comfortable. If he begins to fuss for no reason you can put your finger on, if he loses some of his nice rosy-cheeked color, he may be getting chilly.

Blankets on his crib? You may prefer a sleeping bag, appropriate in warmth to the temperature of the sleeping room. As soon as babies become mobile at all, they seem to delight in wriggling out from under covers. Sleeping bags are made in varying weights appropriate for the seasons of the year. Sleeping bags can't be kicked off either, and you'll soon find that your young one is quite a kicker (that's how he gets his exercise, kicking and waving his arms about). In warm weather (or if the room in which he's napping is warm) all baby needs is a light covering or a cotton sleeping bag. You don't sleep under heavy covers in hot weather and neither should he.

In any event, blankets—sheets, too—should be large enough to tuck well under the mattress. So should waterproof sheets and covers—or, alternatively, they may be clamped in place with special clamps made for this purpose so that they don't bunch up as the baby moves about. The mattress itself should be flat and firm enough so that the baby is not lying in a "hammock" in the center of it.

HOW ABOUT FRESH AIR?

Being out in the fresh air is good for you, good for older children, good for baby, too. Fresh air, especially cool fresh air, tones up the body, makes a person feel great—full of energy—and stimulates the appetite. All these apply to baby as well as to the rest of the family.

Two or three hours outdoors a day in reasonable weather—that means not snowing, not raining, not far below freezing temperature—is what many doctors recommend for a baby, particularly during the time of year when the house is heated. Dry, hot air dries the inside of the nose and throat and makes baby uncomfortable, just as it does you.

Sunshine? By all means, but go slowly. Of course you'll expose baby to a warm sun only briefly the first time and increase the exposure very gradually—a bad sunburn is just as dangerous as a burn from fire. And even when baby's skin has taken on a pretty, golden tan, you won't leave him in the direct sunlight for a long time, as too much sunshine may be bad for his skin. When you put baby outside to sleep, don't leave him in the direct sun or in a place that will be getting direct sun before you pick him up again. But that doesn't mean no sunshine—it just means, as in everything else, moderation.

A baby who weighs ten to twelve pounds can begin to be exposed to direct sunshine for brief periods when the weather is warm. Bear in mind, too, that bright light in his eyes is annoying—and may be harmful—to baby, so when you expose his face to the sun, place him so that the sun is over the back of his head. That way, his eyebrows will shade his eyes a bit.

How long is "long enough"? Two minutes is ample the first time and add two minutes a day—one minute on his back, one on his stomach. Half an hour is plenty of total time in the direct sunshine even when baby has been gradually accustomed to it in two-more-minutes-each-day doses. And remember—the redness of sunburn doesn't show up right way, so you can't tell by the color of baby's skin whether he's getting too much sun. The redness of a burn doesn't show up until a couple of hours later—too late.

When there is very bright sunshine—such as when you take baby on his first trip to the beach, for example—keep him in the shade the entire time. Even so, there is enough reflected light to give him a burn unless you are careful. When sunbathing the baby in very hot weather, put him on the floor or the ground—on a pad, of course—where he can be cooled by the movement of the air. Down in a carriage or bed, where the sides obstruct the movement of air, he can become overheated.

IS BABY GETTING ENOUGH SLEEP?

The answer to that is probably yes—most babies sleep as much as they need to, with the possible exception of a colicky baby. How much is enough is another question. Again, don't compare your baby to Johnny Jones down the street. Just because Johnny's a sleepyhead and can hardly stay awake long enough to tuck away his dinner doesn't mean that your baby should act the same way. One baby may sleep most of the time, another may spend periods awake being sociable. If everything else seems to be going well, if he's eating his food and seems to be digesting it properly, there's no cause for worry no matter which kind of baby yours turns out to be. Of course, the older the baby gets, the less time he will spend sleeping.

In the early months, the average baby sleeps through from one feeding to the next. As he gets older, he'll sleep less —perhaps he'll have a wakeful period in the late afternoon, then gradually at other times during the day. He'll develop a pattern—asleep at certain times, awake at others—that he will probably repeat each day, little by little cutting down on the sleeping times and adding a little to the wakeful ones.

A lot of what establishes these habit patterns depends on you. Take it for granted that baby will sleep after each feeding, put him down and expect him to sleep, and he probably will.

It's worth repeating—baby doesn't need absolute silence for sleeping unless you unfortunately make him think he does. If you shut off the radio, close doors silently, tiptoe about when he's a newborn, he'll accustom himself to that kind of silence when he's asleep. Then, later, when it's necessary to make a little noise, the slightest sound will waken him. Start him off on the right foot—expect him to sleep through the ordinary noises of household activity and he will get used to doing so.

You'll be making for good sleep habits if you put the baby down to sleep at the same times each day and in the same place. Then he'll get the idea that he's supposed to go to sleep and drift off without fuss. If, as soon as he's finished each feeding, you change him, then put him into his own bed, say something like, "Go to sleep now" and leave the room, he'll get the idea—and at a much younger age than you'd imagine. Of course, when he's a newborn, you'd follow this routine anyway, for newborns spend virtually all their time eating or sleeping. But as the months go by, try to adhere to this pattern: meal, change, to bed without company in the room with him. It will allow you to establish a rhythm to your housework and your own rest, and both you and baby will be the better for it.

BABIES ARE SUCH EARLY RISERS!

Babies, as you will quickly find out immediately after you're home from the hospital, like to get up at the crack of dawn. You may have a brief respite before you begin to omit the 2 A.M. feeding, at which point baby is likely to waken at 6 A.M.—you'll be lucky if it isn't 5!—and demand food. However, when they get to be about six months old, many babies are content to stay asleep, go back to sleep or amuse themselves a bit in the mornings—say, until seven or eight—if you help them to learn this good habit.

How? By not bounding out of bed and rushing to the baby the first time he opens his mouth in the morning. Wait a bit. Let him fuss a little, and he may very well go back to sleep or get interested in something else—his mobile or his baby gym that is strung across his crib, with things to push and pull and play with. Of course, if his fussing changes to insistent—and angry (you'll soon be able to tell from the sound of his voice when he's good and mad)—crying, you won't leave him to "cry it out." There was a period when crying it out was considered good for baby, but we've passed that stage and the best pediatric advice nowadays says that it's wrong to ignore a baby who is really crying for a certain length of time. So you'll get up and feed him. But keep trying. He'll soon get the idea and give you and your husband a bit longer to sleep in the morning.

Another habit of which to break the baby at about six months of age is sleeping in the same room with you and your husband. Of course you may have had him in a separate room all along—if so, this is not a problem. But if you let the baby sleep in your room until, say, he's a year old, you're going to have trouble getting him used to the idea of sleeping in another room. At six months, he's not too "set in his ways" —you can move him elsewhere and he will probably hardly notice the difference, almost certainly not object to it. So change his sleeping room—even if, in a small apartment, this requires a major upheaval and much shifting about of furniture. You'll be glad you did.

A habit better never to get into than to try to get out of is taking the baby into your bed with you. In the first place, nobody will get much sleep—you and your husband will worry about one of you rolling on the baby, and the baby, unused to these surroundings, will be wakeful. But that is not the worst of it: if you get into the habit of taking baby into bed with you, he will get into the habit of *being* in bed with you, and it's a very hard habit to break. He'll consider it a treat—it isn't, not for anyone concerned—and won't be satisfied with anything less.

If he cries, you'll be better off getting up and attending to his needs—changing him, feeding him, perhaps talking to him a few minutes in a quiet voice—and then going back to bed, hoping your visit and attention will have satisfied him. Bear this in mind: taking a baby into his parents' bed is one of the hardest habits to break. If you start it, you may have a child in your bed every morning for years or go through a traumatic experience for both you and the child, trying to break him of the habit. Here's one instance where the best advice, in one word, is: *don't*.

WHY DO BABIES CRY?

Babies cry to make their presence felt, their needs known—they have no other way.

You'll be wondering about it—and worrying about it— the early weeks you are home alone with your first newborn. You ask yourself if he's hungry, if he needs changing, if he has indigestion, if—heaven forbid!—he's coming down with something. Sometimes it's one answer, sometimes another— and sometimes there seems to be no answer at all, and that's normal, too. Very young babies, between the time they are about two weeks old and the time they reach about the age of three months, are getting used to being in the world. Their miraculous little bodies are getting adjusted to being alive. So sometimes they cry for no reason that you can put a name to.

There's an old-fashioned word my mother used to use that covers the situation nicely: fretful. There will be times when your baby is fretful. You'll make sure he's all right—not wet, not hungry, not sick—but he'll still be fretful for a short, and sometimes not so short, period once or several times during the day. Don't worry about it. He's just getting used to being a person.

Of course, the baby may not be exercising his prerogative to be fretful. If there's some other cause, how do you determine what it is?

He may be hungry. If it's nearly time for his next feeding, that is probably the answer. But even if it's not, he may still be hungry. Perhaps—for some reason known only to him—he took much less than the normal amount at his last feeding. Try feeding him again if he persists in crying for fifteen minutes or so. If this solves the problem—yes, he was hungry.

He may have indigestion. Try bubbling him again, even if you got a satisfactory bubble after his last feeding.

He may be sick, although it's not likely. Young babies do get colds and sometimes intestinal infections, but these show themselves in runny noses and coughs or in loose bowel movements. Otherwise, he's not likely to be sick. However, if he *looks* sick to you, you'll ease your mind by taking his temperature—and if he has a fever, you'll call the doctor and tell him what's happening.

He may need changing. Some babies don't seem to mind a bit having wet or even dirty diapers. Others do. Try changing him and see if that solves the problem.

He may simply be tired. Perhaps he stayed awake longer than usual after his last feeding. Perhaps you had visitors who ooh-ed and aah-ed over him and kept him awake. Just as sometimes it's too cold to snow, sometimes baby is too tired to sleep—at least, he won't sleep without a fretful period which gradually diminishes until he's dropped off to dreamland. If the fretting lasts more than fifteen or twenty minutes and worries you, try putting him to sleep by walking him or rocking him. But don't make a habit of that—if you do, it will become baby's habit never to go to sleep unless he's rocked or walked, and you'll be deeply sorry you started it.

Soon your ear will be tuned to the differences between one cry and another. You'll be able to listen a moment and then say, "He's hungry," or "He needs changing," or "He's got colic," or "He's just mad at the world—he'll get over it." And you do what's necessary—you feed him or change him or you make him as comfortable as you can or you try to jolly him out of his bad mood with a little cuddling and playing. But you don't worry—you'll have learned the "I am sick" tone of his crying and know that only then do you need to do something out of the ordinary, such as taking his temperature and calling the doctor.

HAVE I "SPOILED" MY BABY?

That worries you because you know that nobody much likes a "spoiled brat"—and, authorities say, the spoiled child doesn't really like himself much, either. He may get his way, but he gets it with considerable trouble and he's aware of his parents' disapproval even though they give in. A twelve-month-old tyrant is pretty hard to take—and somehow, he finds himself hard to take, too. So you're doing no one a favor when you spoil your baby by giving him everything he wants and everything you may think he wants.

It's unlikely that a baby three months old or younger can be spoiled. At that age he's probably not aware enough of cause and effect. He can't reason: If I set up a howl, mother will come running so I guess I'll begin to cry.

By the time he's over his colicky period, if he has one, and has passed his three-month birthday, he *can* be spoiled, however. If you think "He's so little, he needs me to do these things," instead of thinking "If I do, I'll spoil him—and nobody, not even baby himself, will like him," you'll probably spoil your baby. But if you adopt the second attitude, things will work out fine.

6

Don't They Grow Fast!

How rapidly babies grow—both mentally and physically! To a watching mother who never misses the merest quiver of her baby's eyelid, he often seems to be growing and changing before her very eyes. It's truly amazing to see their progress. Even when you consider how much they have to learn and how many skills they have to acquire, the first few weeks of your baby's life are so full of steady, surprising achievements that you're likely to end up secretly thinking "There's going to be no stopping this one!" Don't be self-conscious about it—most new parents feel the same way.

THERE'S SO MUCH TO START WITH . . .

From the very beginning, a baby is able to do a great many things. Why, during the first week he can yawn, sneeze, lift his chin and hiccup. He can certainly suck. He can even communicate with you about the things that are most important to him—hunger and discomfort—by yelling his head off. In a way he can show anger, too, though he's really, again, only reacting to discomfort. If you don't think so, try holding his head in order to guide him toward the nipple of breast or bottle. Not just touching it, but holding it steady. You'll see at once from the way he pulls away that he doesn't care for the restraint.

By the end of the first month, his eyes will follow a moving object. His ears are alert to many kinds of sounds. His whole body will jerk in response to a loud, sharp noise. Offer him a finger—his tiny hand will grip it like a vise. His taste buds, too, are beginning to develop. They will react to sweet, sour, bitter and salty tastes. He has already learned, through his skin sensations, a great deal about the distress of cold and pain, of the pleasure of warmth and cuddling, of pleasant-feeling textures.

Of course these are all reflex actions. He doesn't do them on purpose—"because he wants to"—and he has no control over them. But they do pave his way toward the voluntary actions that will come later. As his muscle control improves and his central nervous system develops, he will start to do many more things intentionally. With this reflex activity, his body is practicing for its future development.

HOW MUCH DO THEY SEE?

Like most young mothers, when my children were infants, I wondered just how much they could see, and felt quite convinced that the authorities who claimed they saw very fuzzily were wrong. My babies certainly knew me! At that time, however, the doctors believed that newborn babies couldn't focus their eyes enough to see clearly, so that all they saw was a kind of blur. I was delighted when more advanced studies showed that all the time mothers like me had been right—no matter what the authorities had said. Nobody has yet gone so far as to claim that when your month-old infant follows you with his eyes, it's because he knows you're his mother—but most authorities do feel that a one- or two-month old is responding to a human face and to the sense of comfort and security he already associates with it.

And, of course, he smiles, as every mother knows. It's all right nowadays to call that charming expression a smile. They (those outdated authorities again) used to try to tell us that it was nothing but an accidental grimace probably caused by a gas bubble. But these days it's accepted as the real thing—a genuine expression of joy and welcome with which your baby suddenly one day rewards you. It's real enough so that researchers at a nationally-known infant behavior study institute are doing research on the smiles of babies, incidentally, and they've come up with one odd bit of news that the Women's Liberation people aren't going to be as happy about as are the mothers of girl babies. Girls, it seems, smile more frequently than boys, and the researchers are investigating the possibility that this may be because they're more anxious to please.

RESPONDING TO OTHER FACES

When your baby begins turning his head to follow your movements around the room, he will also begin to respond to other faces. Very fast progress is made during those first weeks in his ability to recognize not only parents, or those who are always around, but other important people in his life. There seems to be an especially close interaction here between this ability to notice and recognize and the amount of mothering a baby receives. The more time and close, warm attention a mother is able to give her child at this stage, the more rapidly his visual education appears to develop. Perhaps as she holds him and talks to him, she helps to direct his attention to the little world around him.

In any case, by the time he's six months old he's recognizing people from clear across the room. He's looking at himself, too, discovering fingers and toes and other parts of his body, though it's possible that when he first notices something as far away as his own foot, he's somewhat like a kitten that's just noticed its tail—not at all sure that this strange object is attached to him!

Quite often, a baby will have one eye that turns inward or outward and doesn't focus with the other. This is another one of those things not to worry about. He looks, temporarily, cross-eyed, but all he's got is something many babies have at one time or another in their early weeks—strabismus. It's due to a weak muscle, and almost always it corrects itself as the baby matures. However, call your doctor's attention to it. He'll keep tab on it, and if it persists for longer than he thinks it should—which would probably be when the baby is more than six months old—he'll know what to do about it.

Also, don't worry if your baby has something in his eye—a bit of fluff, say, from his blanket—and doesn't appear to notice it. It doesn't mean he's blind or has some nonworking nerves. A small baby's eyes are—to us, very strangely—insensitive. He just isn't bothered by a piece of foreign matter.

CHANGING ATTITUDES

By the way, be prepared as baby gets up into the five- and six-month stage for a new development in his attitude toward the rest of the world. Here you've got this delightfully smiling, outgoing, cuddly little human being and suddenly one day he looks up at a new face—and there's no smile. In fact, he freezes, and when his little face again begins to show emotion, it's the wrong kind—he wails. What's happened is that you have a sensitive, very observant baby who's now gathered enough experience to be able to tell the strange and new from the familiar. And if strange things, places or people scare him a little, that's to be expected. If your mother-in-law suggests you've gone amiss somewhere and made your child overly tense, tell her—politely—that she's quite wrong and that he's only going through a normal stage.

As we said earlier, the baby's hearing comes along quickly, too. You'll realize that the day the front door accidentally slams—and in his crib upstairs your baby's whole body jerks in response. What if it doesn't, which to you means there's something wrong with his hearing? Well, if he's only two or three weeks old, mention it to your doctor but don't worry about it. Babies are born with a certain amount of excess fluid in their ears which prevents them from hearing during their first days. Normally this fluid is absorbed quite quickly, but in some babies the process takes longer—perhaps a few weeks—and during this time the mother may be afraid there is a hearing problem. Your doctor will probably be able to reassure you on that score as soon as you tell him about it—but again, he'll keep an eye on it and know if it's lasting longer than usual.

You can communicate a lot with your baby through his awareness of sound. Music, for instance—its ability to soothe or stimulate him—is well known to any mother who has ever sung her baby a lullaby or asked someone to turn down a lively piece of music that was keeping him awake. You'll see an alert baby kick and rock in time—sometimes in very good time, which is always rather a comical thing to watch—when he hears peppy music. Change it to a slow, lower-keyed number and observe how he's lulled by it. You'll learn something from this about what makes a good lullaby.

THE LULL IN LULLABIES

People who haven't actually sung lullabies to babies are sometimes critical of what seems to them to be the "monotony" of lullabies, both words and music—but people who *have* sung them to babies are a lot more understanding. You have to remember that the whole objective of a lullaby is to get baby to go to sleep. It's not supposed to be a display of your singing talent. If the tune is too entertaining, and if there are sharp or hard sounds in the words that catch his attention (even though he's not listening for meanings, yet), then your lullaby isn't going to work the way you want it to. What you're after is a nice, monotonous, droning song. If the words are repetitious, too, then you've got a working lullaby that's ideal for your purpose.

Lullabies needn't be confined to just music. Other sounds can prove to be just as soothing—and what a blessing this can be when you're busy and can't sit and croon to him, and he just won't seem to go off to sleep by himself. Many young mothers who have taken the time to experiment—maybe they were a little desperate because their babies had the kind of temperamental makeup that made it hard for them to relax and drift off—have told me that a variety of household sounds can be used to put their particular babies to sleep.

Stubborn ones often submit beautifully to the persistent sound of running water, the drone of a vacuum cleaner, the hum of a hair dryer. If you can't turn your back on household tasks and just sit down to sing your resisting one to sleep, arrange the chores so that one of those sounds will substitute for your voice at the right time. Try them. If they don't work, do your own experimenting. It could end with your husband coming home to find you've cut the grass because you've discovered that the lawn mower provides your particular baby with the perfect lullaby. Experiment on your own!

Leaving lullabies aside, there are all kinds of sounds that your baby will find extremely interesting. Which means they'll be educational, too. Try a music box, record player or radio. And don't confine yourself to music. Let him listen to words—a news broadcast, a play. This can accomplish one of two good things. You'll accustom him both to voices and words that he doesn't hear around him all day long. And if they don't happen to catch his attention, they might have the fringe benefit of getting him used to sleeping while something's going on around him. As I said before, keeping your home dead quiet so baby can sleep is rather unwise. Too often this leads to a baby who's fretful and unhappy when you're having company.

A baby who's used to having sounds around him that aren't always familiar is more likely to go to sleep and to keep on sleeping right through your company's conversation. This serves to remind you that even though you're a mother, it doesn't mean you stop being a social person who has a perfect right to sit down and enjoy a conversation with friends. Besides, you're sure to enjoy the conversation more because there may be comments on what a good baby you have!

NOW WE'RE MOVING!

No two babies develop at quite the same rate. Everyone has surely told you that already, and told you more than once. Of course there are general guides about when the average baby, if there is such a thing, is likely to start doing this or that. If you talk it over with your doctor, you'll quickly realize that at least half a dozen things have to be considered in evaluating a baby's progress—mostly, the baby himself.

It's a big, complicated subject, but what it adds up to right now is that if your baby isn't doing at four or five months exactly what the baby next door is doing, it doesn't mean something's wrong with yours or the fellow next door is smarter. It just means they're two *different* people—which, if you stop to think about it, you already know. Each of them is going to come along at his own rate and in his own way, no matter what anyone tells you about what's "average."

But, just in general, at three or four months, your baby

will become aware of what his fingers can do. Amazing! They're tasty. He can suck them (he already knows all about that) and chomp on them with hard little gums that are already beginning to bother him a bit because of the teeth that will soon be coming. And they send messages to him when he uses them for feeling. They've already told him a lot about where his toes and his nose are and what his toys and his clothes feel like. Then at four or five months his muscles start working better and he can grasp those toys. As he goes on toward six and seven months, the coordination between hand and eye improves so that when he grabs an object, it's on purpose, and he can bring it up to where he wants it. Can you imagine how powerful this makes him feel?

Yes, but there he goes again, reaching for his rubber duck with his left hand! He did the same thing a minute ago. Why not his right hand—does this mean he's going to be left-handed? The answer to that is it's too early to tell, and you can't make a judgment, nor can your doctor, from the fact that he happens just now to be using his left hand as much as his right. The best research we have up to now seems to show that some babies use both hands interchangeably during the first year and then gradually start using one—generally the right—more often than the other. Some babies start out concentrating on one hand and then change over to concentrate on the other. Fewer start out with a preference for one hand—again, it's generally the right—and never change back.

What you can do (besides not worrying) is to sort of keep an eye on your baby's habits. There's nothing wrong with left-handedness. It's just an inconvenience in a right-handed world—but if it's an inconvenience you'd just as soon spare him, try in a completely casual way to encourage him to reach for things with his right hand. Offer him his toys at an angle that makes his right hand the logical one for him to reach out with. But never make a big thing out of it. If he reaches with the left hand, give him the toy anyway. If you check with your doctor, he'll probably confirm that medical science really doesn't know for certain whether left-handed babies are born that way or for some reason develop that way, but whichever it is, it's not a thing that matters a lot.

My best friend when I was about fourteen was a left-handed girl, and she used to point out that her left-handed father managed to hand out a bigger allowance for her with his left hand than my right-handed father did for me. (We stayed friends anyway.) Stay relaxed. Your baby's probably going to settle down with his right hand sooner or later, and if he doesn't what of it?

YOUR BABY, THE ATHLETE

Around the age of six months, more or less, baby will perform a fabulous feat—he'll roll over. Big as that rolling-over day is, it's nothing compared to the day he sits up alone for the first time. This, again, is a more-or-less period—anywhere from perhaps six months to nine months or so. If you think about it, you can see how much the time element has to depend on the particular baby. If he's a plump one and tends to go at everything thoughtfully and carefully, he's likely to take longer. If he's skinny and tough and pushy, he'll probably give it a try somewhat earlier.

You'll know, because when you hold out your hands, you'll feel him trying to use them to pull himself up. When he seems to mean it, you can prop him up against a good-sized pillow that supports his back and neck in as straight a position as possible. But watch him. Those little back muscles are still weak. You can't leave him up there like that for very long. The moment he starts showing the least sign of fatigue, down he goes again. The signs to watch for are slumping forward, curling up or sliding down on the small of the back. Sometimes they seem to say, "I've had enough of this for now!" by simply toppling over sideways—there's no mistaking that.

When he can sit up against a pillow for any length of time, he's ready for a wider world than he's had up to now in his nursery. Give him a change of scene by moving him into the room you're going to be in for a time. Put him in a car seat or his stroller or at his feeding table, if you have one, and let him *supervise your work—he'll enjoy it. But again—don't let him* stay up too long. Even if he doesn't start slumping he may become fretful, and that's probably a signal that he'd welcome a new position.

Are you ready for crawling? Because pretty soon *he* will

be—and that's another landmark day! Crawling is a wonderful form of exercise, for it uses nearly every muscle in baby's little body. Generally, the ball-of-fire babies will begin this stunt at an earlier age than the placid ones will, but by the time it happens (six months to a year), you'll already have some feeling for your baby's particular pattern and pace of development, so if he's a late crawler, you won't be fretting over his slowness. He isn't slow; he's just *him,* crawling when *he's* ready.

It's amazing how many crawling styles there are. Some babies start out crawling backward. Some crawl sideways. Some go on hands and toes without bending their knees, so that their legs are straight and their little bottoms are the highest part of them. There's another interesting variation where a baby combines two methods—using one knee and keeping the other leg straight.

Don't fret about it if your baby is clumsy at first, even though he seems to think he's ready. In no time he'll probably be scooting around so fast you'll get into the habit of looking down every time you take a step—he's likely to be under it! And don't worry even if he doesn't get around to crawling at all. There are some babies who bypass this stage altogether. It often seems as though it's the noncrawlers, or the awkward crawlers, who start walking early, while the expert, speedy crawlers are a little less eager to get up and start walking. After all, they're getting around just fine on hands and knees or hands and toes.

THE REAL MIRACLE—WALKING

Before walking, of course, comes standing. There's always the little eager beaver who pulls himself up when he's perhaps six or seven months old. At whatever age, he'll be so pleased with himself and with this new skill that he won't want to sit down. Of course there's also the little problem that he can't exactly handle—*how* to sit down. But it's perfectly true that, overcome with the glory of the achievement, most babies don't want to cut it short.

Sometimes a baby will stand and stand until you can see he's frantic with exhaustion, yet when he's unhitched from the playpen railings and lowered, he'll scream with anger and haul himself back up. The best solution I've found to this problem is to give baby something especially intriguing to play with when you sit him back down—perhaps something you've saved for the purpose so that its newness will be surefire. And comfort yourself with the thought that he's done the hard part; within a week he'll probably have figured out how to sit back down by himself. Sitting-down day is another of the big days—a bigger day for you, perhaps, than for him.

Now, having learned to stand and sit, his next step—and that's literally what it is—is to move about his playpen. He does it cautiously, and it's quite fascinating to watch. First he hangs on with both hands and pushes a foot forward. After a while he holds on with only one hand. Then he lets go altogether. He's standing on his own two feet. Look, Mommy, no hands!

UP—AND COMPLETELY FREE

Many different things will decide the age when a baby actually walks alone (usually a better way to say it would be "totter" alone, because even the most determined walker isn't going to start out with a firm, measured tread but something more like a series of lurches). As I said, how well he crawls may have a lot to do with it. Illness can affect it. A sick spell when he's just beginning to walk may delay progress for several weeks, even though the illness itself is quite trivial and brief. And don't underestimate the discouraging effect of falling down.

If you put yourself in your baby's place—and it's not easy—you'll begin to appreciate what it means to this small, tender, protected creature to have nothing to lean against, nothing to support him, nothing to hang on to—there he stands, completely free for the first time in his life, but also completely without support.

A fall from this magnificently upright position may not hurt him in the least—generally he just sort of folds up and plops—but to him it can be a bad experience. Don't be surprised if a little topple that looks like nothing to you frightens baby into going back to clinging to you or the furniture or the playpen bars, or even back to crawling. After all, that's a tried and trusted method, and he did get to see things. He'll get up again in a little while. Don't force it. Be very patient.

A few extra-lively babies may start to walk as early as nine months. Some perfectly bright and healthy ones stall around until they're as old as a year and a half. They simply aren't in any rush, that's all. If we have to fix on an average—that worrisome word again—most doctors would tell us twelve to fifteen months. The big thing is that your baby will walk when he's ready. His muscular development, his sense of balance, the degree of self-confidence he's built up from all his earlier triumphs—all these, plus his weight and strength, are going to make the decision. Don't fall for that old-fashioned idea that if a baby starts to walk too early, he'll have bowlegs or knock-knees. He can't start "too early" because if it's too early, he won't start.

LOUD AND CLEAR

And now about talking. Your baby is actually learning to talk long before you can pick words out of his babbling. When he's very young, you'll already see that he understands and responds to certain words that have meaning for him, and many of the sounds he himself makes are, in a sense, words. When he responds over and over with a particular sound to you or his food or his bath or a special toy, he's using words, even though nobody can find them in any dictionary. Some babies lie there and gurgle and chirp and babble to themselves at a great rate—and often if you listen very closely, you'll be able to pick what seems like a real word out of the stream of sounds.

But generally you can't look for this until he's around a year old. Some perfectly bright, normal children don't do any real talking until they're two; some even wait until they're three. This isn't average, so your doctor should be alerted. But when a late talker finally does start, the chances are he'll come out with complete sentences. He was just biding his time until he was good and ready.

Now—granted that you've got the normal, healthy baby you almost certainly have—talking is a social accomplishment. It can be affected a great deal by you and the other people who have a lot of contact with him—by how much *you* talk to *him,* by the way you talk, by the atmosphere you create, and by many other things. If he's talked at, or talked to, too much he may freeze up. It's almost as though you're not giving him a chance to get a word in edgewise.

If you talk to your baby gently, with affection, form your words clearly, don't use too many of them—no long sentences—and watch how he responds, you'll soon get a sort of feel of your own for the best way to start reaching him with language. Try to use the same word for the same thing each time you bring it up. His kitty may also be named Tommy, but if you point to it once and say *kitty,* and the next time you say *Tommy*—well, put yourself in the baby's place. It's more than a little confusing to someone who's just starting to learn to use any words at all.

Feeding time is a particularly good time to talk to baby. He sees the same few objects over and over again at every meal—bottle, dish, spoon and so on. And they're intensely important to him. I wouldn't try to introduce him to "strained peas" or "beef stew"; just "food" might be a better word for all of it. "Here's your spoon," in the right, easy, pleasant tone, could have your baby saying "spoon" before you realize he's said it. Of course what comes out the first time around might be "poo." Don't make a big joke out of it, and don't make "poo" the household word for spoon forever after because it was baby's first word. Your baby isn't talking baby talk to be cute; he's doing his best to come out with what you've said even though he hasn't quite made it yet. Help him by repeating that it's a *s*poo*n*—treat him with a little respect.

There's nothing in the world more fascinating than watching your baby grow and develop from his very first days. Don't treat him as something only to be cared for and waited on. He's a person, not a doll or a pet, and you have to communicate with a person to get to know him. Find as much time as you can to be with him, talk to him, play with him; share his experiences. Be there to see his face when he finally pulls himself up on his feet. See the world through his eyes—you haven't had a chance like that since *you* were in the playpen, and at that point you really didn't know what was going on! So—enjoy the experience.

7

Babyproof the Place

Much of the charm of very small children lies in their vulnerability. Babies, in their innocence, are ignorant of the hazards of life. It's up to the adults to think ahead to protect them from their own ignorance and curiosity and from the accident situations in the world around them.

A study made by the federal government's Department of Health, Education and Welfare shows that every year children under fifteen suffer almost 16.5 million injuries from accidents—and that nine out of ten of these injuries need not have happened if elementary precautions and ordinary common sense had been exercised. Most accidents don't just "happen"—the groundwork for them is laid by carelessness, by thoughtlessness.

You'll have to train yourself to be safety-conscious, not just in dangerous situations but all the time, for what, to you, can be ordinary circumstances holding no peril can be extremely dangerous situations for a baby. You wouldn't for example, stick a wire into an electric outlet. You know better. But baby does not know any better, and he may very well get a bad shock if you don't cover unused wall plugs.

Where will baby find a wire? How about a hairpin or bobby pin accidentally dropped on the floor?

THINK-SAFETY HABIT

You'll learn the think-safety habit so that it becomes second nature to you—learn, for example, to pick up immediately everything you drop, to run a quick eye around the room periodically to see what's left out or misplaced or otherwise changed so that it creates a hazard.

Of course baby's safe until he can crawl freely around the room, until he begins to stand upright and walk a little? Wrong. There are hazards to be dealt with almost from the moment he joins the family. These are not as many as those he'll encounter as he grows a bit and learns new skills, but the time to begin to think safety every minute is when he's very small so that you'll develop the habit.

What can harm a small baby? His own crib, for example, if you leave him alone in it with the crib sides down—even for a moment. Even the quietest baby, once he's old enough to turn over by himself, is in danger in such a situation— he may roll, roll again and fall out. Don't leave baby untended on a big bed, either. He hasn't yet learned to roll over? Never mind—you might leave him at exactly the moment he's about to learn this trick that babies love so much! Even if he can't roll, he can wiggle and wriggle to the edge and fall off. Never allow this situation to occur, and you'll never have occasion to be sorry that you did.

Somehow it seems impossible to ignore a ringing telephone or doorbell—but you'll have to learn to do just that when baby is in the bathtub, his own or the grown people's tub. Left alone for a second—even long enough for you to cross the room to get the soap you forgot—baby can come to harm in a bathtub. He can fall out of a small plastic tub, for example. He can slide underwater in almost any tub. He can slip and hit his head against the hard sides. Even in a bathinette there's still the water to be thought of. If you simply can't ignore the phone or bell, scoop baby up into a towel and take him along.

While we're on the subject of bathing, don't forget to test the bath water with your elbow before putting baby into his bath. And if you're bathing him in the sink, bathroom basin or big tub, remember to turn off the hot-water faucet before you turn off the cold if you have a mixer faucet; or turn the hot one off a few moments before you put baby into the tub. With that precaution, the little head and flailing small arms never come in contact with a faucet that is painfully hot.

Those are the chief little-one hazards. But you'll find, as I did, that when baby learns to crawl, then to stand and inch himself around by hanging on to things, then finally to walk by himself—that is the time when the possibilities for accidents multiply so rapidly it's hard to keep up with them. The toddler's ambition in life seems to be to wriggle off of, climb into, up to, onto and down from everything in sight and to put everything possible (and a number of things you wouldn't believe possible) into his mouth or his nose or his ears!

Fortunately, most accidents that small children have are minor ones, resulting only in skinned knees and bumped heads. Even so, all of us mothers have to keep in mind that the bad accident is possible if we're not ever watchful, for such accidents kill more children than all the seven most common diseases of childhood put together.

A LIST OF HAZARDS

As soon as baby shows the first signs of creeping, go through the house and do a complete putting-away job. For the time being, find new, high-up or locked-up places for everything that might harm baby and everything that you cherish, even though it might do baby no harm—babies have a certain kinship to a horde of locusts when it comes to ruining things.

Put out of baby's reach ashtrays, vases, framed pictures, bibelots, sculpture. Take all the books off low shelves—babies love their own books to look at and the big people's to chew on! Magazines, too, will have to go up to some high place. Hobby and other needlework materials should be put away—preferably in a room (where they can be worked on) that has a lock on the door. If daddy brings work home from the office, warn him that it will likely get chewed unless he puts it safely away the moment he's through with it. True, your house may look a bit unlived-in—or, at least, pretty top-heavy—but you'll thank your stars a hundred times that you made every effort to babyproof the place.

What other hazards are there? Plenty! Take a look at baby's high chair, for example. Is it spread-legged, broad at the base, so that he can't tip it over when he goes into his gymnastics while sitting in it? Do you have a harness to hold him in it so he can't fall out? Has the tray a safety latch to keep him from pulling it into the up position? Never leave baby alone in a room in his highchair—even with harnesses babies have slipped between chair and tray and been seriously injured.

Windows in a house or apartment can be dangerous. Anything higher than the first floor should have guards or never be opened except from the top. (Actually, I'd do the same with ground-floor windows, just to be absolutely sure!)

Stairs seem to offer creepers and toddlers a special challenge. Unlike older people, little explorers find it easier to get up the stairs than down—they'll manage to get up and then are stranded at the top like the kitten that has climbed too high in a tree. (Fortunately you don't have to send for the fire department, as with kittens.)

The thing to do is to forestall any climbing by protecting stairs—both top and bottom—with gates. Perhaps your husband can make these, or they can be purchased at hardware stores or stores specializing in items for children. While you're babyproofing stairs, don't forget the porch steps if you have any.

MORE GROWING-UP PAINS

The kitchen is filled with hazards. Indeed, there's so much danger of spilling hot water or oil or foods that it's safest never to allow the baby to crawl around the kitchen when you're working there. If he's in the kitchen with you, put baby in his high chair, where he can enjoy your company and you can talk to him and give him the metal measuring spoons—for some reason children just love them—to play with. Or bring the playpen up to the door of the kitchen and let baby watch you from that vantage point.

But even if you promise yourself never to let the baby creep or toddle around the kitchen when you're working, get into the habit of turning pot handles out of reach, all the same. That's for insurance. You'll get so you do it automatically, and that will be wise—you're often in some other part of the house while you leave things cooking on the stove.

And get into another habit—take a swift look around the kitchen before you leave. Have you left out anything that baby might get later—knives or cookie cutters or anything else with sharp edges on a table or counter that he can reach? (Don't forget that one of the things a toddler learns early is to pull a chair or stool over and climb up on it to help him reach—early training for later raids on the cookie jar, no doubt.) Have you left a garbage can where he can rummage through its contents—one that may at best have dirty food in it, at worst broken glass or cans with jagged edges?

Are ammonia, washing soda, bleach, wax removers, metal polish, borax, mothballs, lighter fluids, shoe polish all in some place you are absolutely certain the baby can't get into? Have you left a pail of water on the floor? Baby isn't likely to hurt himself on it unless it has sharp places where the handle meets the body—but think of the mess it can create if he knocks it over! Are there foods like peas or beans or nuts that he can put into his mouth and perhaps suck into his throat and choke on or stuff into his ears or nose?

Take one last look around, always! On the same theme, take a look around the living room—have you left out dishes of popcorn, nuts or candy? Is there a letter opener on the desk, a sharp pencil by the telephone? Or, more for your sake than his, are there any magazines around that he can reduce to waste paper in nothing flat? Are there cigarettes anywhere, burning or not? Lighters? Matches? Babies are fantastically quick at reaching and grabbing, at getting into mischief while your back is turned for one split second!

Sometimes I think it isn't safe to give a baby anything smaller than an anvil to play with. Check over his toys—any loose buttons used on clothes or for eyes or nose or mouth? Any loose wheels that he can work off and chew on?

Even if the toy is of pretty good size, will it come apart into smaller pieces?

OTHER SOURCES OF TROUBLE

In the bedroom, is there perfume or toilet water he might drink? Are there pills on nightstands? A wastebasket full of "treasures" for baby to rout through? Manicure implements he might injure himself with? Cosmetics he might decide to sample? In the bathroom, is the medicine cabinet locked? Are discarded razor blades safely disposed of in a can with a narrow slit on top? Is the toilet seat *always* kept closed? Are shampoos, hair tonics and home-permanent liquids safely locked away?

Medicines are another source of trouble. Some of them that adults can take are harmful to young ones even in very small quantities. Others that might be harmless in a small quantity can be lethal in large doses. Aspirin, for example, can be one of the most dangerous of household drugs. For some reason, aspirin seems to appeal to small children. They gobble it as if it were candy—I wonder why, when it's so bitter?—sometimes, if not watched, getting away with the contents of a whole bottle. Many children have died from aspirin poisoning. The smartest thing to do with medicine is to keep it all in a cabinet that is both out of reach and that has a babyproof latch or a lock.

Along the same lines, don't let your toddler see you taking medicine—there's no point in fostering the idea that pills or liquids in bottles, large or small, are for eating or drinking. Take your medicine out of baby's sight and put it back in a safe place as soon as you're through with it. And don't ever coax a child to take medicine by telling him it's candy. Concerning candy, children feel that if some is good, more is better.

THOSE MEDICINES CAN BE POISON!

Don't encourage them to think that way about medicines! Be sure medicines are well labeled so that you won't give the youngster—or any other member of the family—the wrong one. Throw away remains of medicines after an illness is over—you'll be unlikely to use them again, and anyway, many medicines deteriorate. In the ordinary course of things, don't change medicines from their original container to another. An exception to this is the "childproof" container—difficult to open—that you can buy to hold dangerous medicines, especially medicine for the toddler himself.

You'd be surprised at the number of poisonous substances there are around any normal household—and even more, if not strictly poisonous, that could make a child ill if swallowed or inhaled. Detergents, for instance, powdered or liquid. Liquid cleaners, with or without ammonia. Window cleaners. Soaps of various kinds, solid or powdered. Room deodorant sprays. Insecticides of all kinds. Steel wool. Scouring powders. Dishwasher powders and rinses. Dry cleaners for clothing. Furniture cleaners and polishers. The list is practically endless.

Most hardware stores will supply you with doorstops and safety knobs that will prevent the toddler from opening doors he should not open, safety latches and locks for medicine cabinets and kitchen cabinets that are too complicated for small fingers to work, for little minds to figure out.

Here are the things that most often cause serious poisoning in children: aspirin, followed closely by other drugs; insect poisons and rat poisons; lead in paint (usually outdoor paint from such places as windowsills); furniture polish; auto polish; lye; cleaners for drains, toilet bowls and ovens; oil of wintergreen; sprays for plants.

CURIOSITY CAN KILL

Toddlers have very little discrimination, and no matter how horrible a substance may smell, look or taste, a child will sample it, sometimes even consume large amounts of it. So put all such things far out of reach or, better yet, lock them up—and *know* baby's safe from them.

Inspect your house for "danglers," too—things that hang over the edge of other things so that baby's small hands can catch hold and tug and pull the whole kit and kaboodle down on his head. Doilies and table covers and dresser scarves that hang over the edge of the furniture they're protecting are danglers. Plants with trailing stems are danglers. Cords of table lamps are danglers. Anything that looks inviting to pull on is a dangler, and you can be virtually certain that at some point or other it will be pulled on.

Electric cords, besides being arranged in such a way that they are not inviting for small hands to pull on, should be kept in good shape. Never leave a worn cord, its insulation frayed, where baby can get at it. (For the whole family's safety, you shouldn't give such a cord house room, anyway.) Wall outlets not in use should be closed with the special plugs made for that purpose—some present-day outlets close themselves when the plugs are pulled out. Never touch, or allow your young one to touch, electrical equipment while in the bathtub or while using or standing in water or while holding on to a faucet.

HARM OUTDOORS

Just babyproofing the house doesn't get you home free. When you've done everything you can inside, go outdoors. Tools, and especially power tools, must be kept locked away from little hands. A rotary lawn mower is lethal. Deep ditches should be fenced in—or the baby fenced away from the ditches. Don't let a toddler get more than a couple of steps ahead of you, even in your own yard, especially near the street or road.

It's amazing how fleet of foot a small child can turn, even one who was stumbling awkwardly, hardly able to stand up, a moment ago. It goes without saying that wells, pools and cisterns should be well protected, either with sufficiently high walls or with very heavy covers. Even a small plastic "baby" pool can be dangerous—don't leave your toddler splashing alone in one any more than you'd leave him alone in the bathtub.

Never put an insecticide or pesticide into any container other than the one it came in—never into such a thing as a soft-drink bottle, for example. Use—or construct or have constructed, if one can't be adapted—a secure lock-up cabinet for turpentine, paints and paint thinners, kerosene, gasoline, benzene, weed killers, insecticides, antifreeze, car polishes.

If by any chance your young explorer does eat or drink something that is poisonous—and it sometimes does happen despite all your precautions—call the hospital immediately, then get to the emergency room as fast as you can, taking along the container of whatever it was that the youngster ate or drank. The doctor will need to see the label in order to know what sort of antidote to use.

Keep youngsters away from strange dogs and cats or other animal pets until they reach an age when they understand that if they hurt the animal it may retaliate. Be careful even with family pets, particularly small ones that are easily hurt. Quite innocently, toddlers will pull tails, yank ears, stick fingers in eyes. The baby should be protected from the pet, the pet from the baby.

NOT TOO MUCH FUSS, PLEASE

Babies learning to walk will fall down, but they seldom hurt more than their pride, so try not to make a fuss. Check for damage, of course, but it's a good idea to stay matter-of-fact, even cheerful, so that baby won't become overly apprehensive about falls. If you apparently take small accidents in your stride, he will, too.

By the way, I've found that when babies do have accidents and are screaming, yet there is no blood or other visible sign of injury, it's wise to offer a toy, cookie or a piece of candy. If that will distract baby and turn off the tears, he was more frightened than hurt. If he refuses to be distracted, then you can start to worry.

When you take your youngster along to do the shopping, you'll need to keep an especially close watch on him in the shopping cart, for babies have a positive genius for grabbing the middle can in a pyramid and sending the rest of the stack toppling over on you. Those quick little hands may add considerably to your grocery bill, too, by picking up gum, razor blades and various other small items when you aren't watching. Of course, you should never leave him unattended in the shopping cart, even momentarily, while you go back a few steps to get some item you'd overlooked. Your toddler can easily send the cart rolling.

Leaving him unattended in the cart outside the market can be still more hazardous, for if the cart starts rolling, it may easily run off a curb and topple over. Don't leave him unattended in buggy or stroller, either, for the same reasons and because, unfortunately, there are in this world disturbed people—generally, frustrated would-be mothers—who might seize the opportunity to take your little one away with them.

Your automobile is another place to be extra specially watchful, since your little one may decide to imitate you and try his hand at driving—and it's so very easy to twist the key if it's left in the ignition or to move the gear shift. Push-button window controls are another hazard if put in operation when a head or an arm is stuck out the window. Those push buttons are very tempting to your young explorer, too!

PRECAUTIONS WHEN DRIVING

Speaking of automobiles and small children, it's wise to use some form of safety belt or harness. An infant's car bed is a safe and comfortable way for a baby to ride; you should place it so that one end will rest on the back seat while the other end of it is secured to the back of the front seat, not laid along the length of the seat. When the baby reaches the toddler stage, a well-constructed car seat is best, with the youngster securely fastened in. The height of the child determines when he can safely use a car seat. A too-short child will slip down in the seat and might be seriously injured if an accident occurs. In a car seat, a youngster large enough to use one is protected during sudden stops and turns, and *you* are protected against his "helping" you drive.

Items of all sizes, from small tacks to clothing home from the cleaners, are packaged in plastic bags, and those bags can be dangerous to children, for a small child can suffocate in one in only a matter of seconds. Accordingly, it's advisable to destroy them or at least to treat them as you do other dangerous substances—lock them away where your youngster can't get to them.

When your youngster begins helping to feed himself, you'll find that plastic dishes and cups are an excellent idea, as many small children consider it a great game to hurl things down. The plastic items not only avoid breakage, they also avoid the danger of your crawling youngster getting broken glass in hands and knees—not to mention keeping the floors safer for the rest of your family.

THE IMPORTANT CHECKLIST

But the old saying, "An ounce of prevention is worth a pound of cure" is as true today as ever. Here's a quick-and-easy checklist to help you make your home safe for baby and for everyone else in the family.

IN GENERAL:

Plastic bags—knot several times before discarding; keep new kitchen bags out of baby's reach.

Toys—don't allow baby to have any smaller than his fist; be sure all buttons, facial features, wheels are securely fastened; don't allow toys with sharp points or edges.

Lighting—be sure all rooms of the house and all corners of the rooms are well lighted; don't leave empty sockets in lamps or fixtures—put a bulb in even if you don't intend to use it.

Rugs—make certain that all large ones lie flat, without turned-up edges for small feet to trip on, that all small ones are anchored securely.

Drawers, cabinet doors, table legs, lamp cords, electric appliances and switches—make sure all are kept in good repair.

Windows—make sure each has a tight screen or storm window or a guard; or, at the least, that windows are opened only from the top.

Stairways—make certain that each has a good handrail; babyproof tops and bottoms of stairs—in house, to basement, to porch—with gates.

IN THE KITCHEN:

Cutlery—have a safe storage place for knives, forks, other pointed or edged kitchen utensils.

Cleaning agents—keep all cleaners and polishes locked up; matches, too.

Floor—wipe up spilled water, spattered grease, spilled food immediately.

Electrical appliances—store in a dry place; make sure cords are in good repair; don't use where baby can pull them down unless constantly supervised.

Stove—keep pot handles turned toward the back of the stove; teach children to stay away from the stove and oven controls—never leave a young one alone near the stove until he's old enough to understand and remember.

IN THE BATHROOM:

Medicines—keep well labeled, store in locked or otherwise tamperproof cabinet.
First-aid kit—keep one in the house, freshly stocked, at all times.
Bathtub and shower—use a nonskid bathtub or shower mat for adults and older children, pad with towel for babies and toddlers.
Plumbing—keep in good repair.

IN THE BEDROOM:

Medicines—don't leave them on night table or other accessible spot.
Cosmetics—keep them safely locked away from toddlers and children.

IN BASEMENT OR GARAGE:

Trash—clear it out!
Tools—keep all away from children; be particularly careful with power tools, mowers.
Poisonous substances—insecticides, pest poisons, plant sprays, paints and thinners should be locked up.

IN THE YARD:

Toys—sliding and climbing toys should be kept in good working order; inspect frequently for loose joints, sharp edges.
Grass—keep it cut to a reasonable length, rake regularly for small rocks, bits of broken glass, sharp sticks.
Garbage can—a "raccoonproof" cover holder is also babyproof.
Tools—return to safe storage immediately after you are through with them.
Porch or patio—if it is high, put a railing around it.

8

The Care and Feeding of Baby-Sitters

No matter what kinds of ideas you have about a mother's place, there are going to be times when someone has to take yours. Even if you're a full-time mother whose whole job is taking care of baby, home and husband, sooner or later you'll need the services of a baby-sitter. And of course if you're planning to be a working mother with a job outside the house—anything from a part-time job that removes you for a couple of afternoons a week to a full-time nine-to-five kind of job—you'll just have to get your hands on a person to whom you can entrust your baby while you're occupied.

THE BEST BABY-SITTER YOU'LL EVER GET

I'd like to pause right here to make a point I think is pretty important. There are baby-sitters . . . and baby-sitters. Someone who comes in for a couple of hours on Friday night so that you and your husband can take in a movie— that's a baby-sitter. But someone who comes in during the day to dress your baby, feed him, play with him, walk him, talk to him, get him down for his nap and be there for him to smile at when he wakes up—that's a mother substitute. If you think about it, they're two different kinds of jobs, and when you're looking for a baby-sitter, it's going to make a difference which of those jobs you're trying to fill.

A few lines back I mentioned your ideas about a mother's place, so maybe I ought to make it plain that I have some of my own. Personally, I favor mothers staying at home with their children except when it's absolutely necessary for them to be away. Naturally when there's a problem of illness or some emergency you don't have a choice, but what I'm talking about are mothers of new babies who tell themselves and everyone else who'll listen that they "can't wait to get back to work."

If you're widowed or divorced or there's real financial need, that's one thing. But if you're working to "fulfill" yourself, it might pay not to make any definite arrangements about your going back to work, or going out to look for a job, until after you've given yourself a chance to investigate the work that's really yours now—mothering. If it's a money question, keep in mind that by the time everything comes out of your paycheck that has to come out of it, there's usually not much left to add to the family budget—hardly enough to make up for what you and your child will lose out of your relationship during his first vital years.

It doesn't make a lot of difference even if you're lucky enough to have someone close—a mother, aunt, sister or friend—who's free and willing to take over for you. However eager she may be, however ready to love and respond to your baby, she's not you—and she's not going to do it just exactly the way you would. And if you have to hire a stranger, it stands to reason that even if you stumbled on the magically perfect person who was made to order for your needs, one prime ingredient wouldn't be there—she wouldn't be your baby's mother.

She might be full of affection for your child and full of interest in his development, but helping him grow into an intelligent, self-confident, open-minded human being wouldn't be identified with her life and personality as it is with yours. Much as child psychologists battle among themselves, there's pretty general agreement among them that during those early years—even the earliest months—the importance of love, security and encouragement can't be overrated. If you're looking for a worthwhile job, can you think of one that could be one-tenth as vitally necessary as supplying those important factors for your own child?

But all of that concerns only the problem of the mother substitute. That's quite different from the custodial care you want from someone who will come in to sit (preferably after baby's tucked in for the night) and answer the phone, listen in case baby cries or—let's face it—pick up the baby and get him outside in case there's a fire. (If there's a chance for her to call the fire department after the baby's safely out, fine, but you want someone intelligent enough to put first things first, don't you?)

HOW AND WHERE TO LOOK . . .

How do you find such a person—or, better still, such people, since the first thing you'll learn as you start looking is that you have to build up a list?

Neighbors and friends are your best bet, particularly those with lists of their own or with teen-agers of their own with whom you already have some acquaintance and who are available for sitting. A relative with time on her hands may save your life on occasion—but as I said, you can't assume that because someone is part of the "family," she's going to be a good person to leave your baby with. People in your own family may have ideas about children quite different from yours.

Other sources you'll find useful are church youth groups, the local YM and YW, 4H clubs if you live in an area that has them and nearby schools, for two reasons—students and teachers. Very often young teachers find night-time baby-sitting a pleasant way to add to their income, for if they're studying for advanced degrees, they can do it as well in your home as in their own and it won't prevent them from being alert to sounds from the nursery. Also, you're getting someone who has already said something about her (or his) attitude toward children—she enjoys them and is interested in them.

High-school guidance departments or the employment

office of a local college will be glad to supply the names of students who want to baby-sit, with the added advantage that you can ask a few questions about the proposed sitter before you meet her yourself. Another good source is a nearby hospital. If you call there, however, be careful to get hold of the right person to talk to. The head nurse's office is likely to think you're asking for a registered nurse to come and baby-sit, and while that would be marvelous in terms of training and experience, the price such a person has the right to ask for her services is not exactly what you have in mind for your evening out.

Ask for social services or the switchboard of the nursing school if there is one. What you want is a student nurse, a well-recommended nurse's aide or even a practical nurse—who's likely to be a responsible, mature woman who likes taking care of people—if there happens to be one available who has the time free that you need. This list of suggestions is only to start you off; as you investigate your own neighborhood, you'll discover local sources that someone who doesn't live there would have no way of knowing about.

... AND WHEN

Don't wait until the day you need a sitter to look for one. First of all, you'll probably find yourself out of luck. Baby-sitting doesn't work that way these days; good baby-sitters are usually lined up weeks in advance for whatever time they have available for the job. Don't forget that this is almost always an activity they squeeze in on top of whatever takes up most of their time—studying or working or caring for their own families or whatever. The one exception to this rule will come from a source I only suggest, for casual baby-sitters, as a last resort—though it might be your first source if what you're going to need is a mother substitute. That's the professional agency. You'll find them either by recommendation or in the Yellow Pages.

But in practical terms this isn't always possible. You've called them because you have an emergency need, and when they send someone out they've pretty much got you over a barrel. You have to accept their candidate because there she is, and your husband is waiting downtown or you have a train to catch, and there isn't time to rethink the whole situation. So off you go leaving your baby with someone who, in all likelihood, is absolutely reliable and honest and sensible —only you don't happen to like her, and you're uneasy all night long and don't have a good time and cut the evening shorter than you meant to. That's no fun, and if you happen to have gone out for some serious or business purpose, it won't enable you to give your full attention to what you have to accomplish, either.

GROUND WORK IS NECESSARY

So—try to meet potential baby-sitters before you're ready to use them and start making yourself a list, with addresses and phone numbers and some notes about how you got the name in the first place, just to remind yourself in case you don't need to call them for some time. Meeting a baby-sitter and having her come into your home and meet your baby are extremely important if you want to do the right thing for everyone concerned. Your reactions are important because you're the adult in charge and it's up to you to set the standards and decide on the needs that come first with *you*.

Maybe that's something you haven't thought about before. Stop to consider it, then, after you talk to your first candidate. If she was a youngster, was she sloppy or terribly far out and mod in dress and/or manner—and if so, does that displease you enough so that you won't want her around your baby? On the other hand, even if her conversation was largely made up of a few words hooked together with "like" and "you know"—"It's like I really dig kids, you know?" is the sort of thing I mean—how did she react to the baby himself? Could you see that she really did "dig" babies? Did she really look at your baby and smile or find a little sound or word for him—without being overeager about it? With a really small baby, her warmth and interest might matter a lot more than her superficial mannerisms.

If it's an older person you're talking to—a grandmother perhaps, with time on her hands for baby-sitting—you may have the opposite problem, someone who's too old or tired to be really interested in your baby. Well, sometimes even that doesn't matter very much. Your first sitters are likely to be left with your baby only after he's asleep for the night, and they won't have anything really to do with him unless there's an emergency or he happens to be wakeful. The sitter won't have to show creative interest, just responsibility and good sense. You have to take that into account, too.

YOU MAKE THE RULES

In both cases, probably the most important thing you have to decide is how sensible and responsible the individual seems. Anyone who's had lots of experience with baby-sitters will assure you that a fourteen-year-old girl who's had a chance to supervise younger brothers and sisters—and who hasn't been turned into a baby-hater by such family-imposed chores!—usually turns out to be a surprisingly efficient baby-sitter, often more so than someone ten or fifteen years older with no experience of caring for young children.

Those are your priorities, then: your reaction of liking or disliking; the impression you get of the individual's sense of responsibility, practical intelligence and—if you can get it —real warmth and interest in babies. Of course to those words about teen-age grooming, which often doesn't meet with your personal standards, I ought to add one point: with a very young baby you want clean clothes and clean hands in the nursery. Don't hesitate to keep on hand a fresh smock—a really "groovy" one won't hurt—and ask your baby-sitter to put it on over her own clothes (you can suggest that it's to protect *them* if you feel awkward about it) when she takes over for the night. Admittedly, it will be easier for you to make this point with a young person than an older one, who's more likely to get huffy. But in either case keep clearly in mind that their feelings are not your primary problem; your baby is. You are entitled to have him handled in the way *you* prefer.

Gracious relations and a sense of all-round warmth and good feeling are terribly important, but not if it means you have to accept something for and around your baby that you don't care for. In any case there's that word "responsibility" again. The right kind of person, no matter what age, is going to understand that your baby—and how you want him handled—comes first in this situation, and she herself won't want to introduce into the nursery any germs or infection that might be avoided.

DO YOUR PART

If your baby-sitting candidate is inexperienced, don't expect too much from her during your "interview"—which should only be an informal, friendly chat—in the way of questions. It's your job to answer the important ones before they're asked. Start an "Information for Baby-Sitters" notebook. Think about it, talk to other mothers about their experiences because there will be things you'll never think of on your own and put all the bases you want to have covered down in the notebook, in clear terms, well before the big occasion when you first leave your baby with someone else.

During your introductory meeting, show the sitter around the house—where baby's clothing and equipment are kept; through your kitchen and refrigerator; where the phones are; where the locks are and how they work; where the fire extinguisher is just in case; the medicine cabinet where she'll find first-aid medication, and anything else you can think of—and then make sure that's all down in writing in your notebook. When she comes to sit, check back again over the most urgent points and show her that she can refer to them again in the notebook. Also into the notebook go the name and phone number of your family physician and that of a nearby friend or relative in case of need.

Introduce her to the family pets, if any, and show her how to approach them. If she doesn't care for animals, try to have them out of the way the night she comes. They're not as important as the baby. Put an emergency list up next to your telephone—the local hospital, police department, fire department, poison control center (you'll hardly need that if your baby isn't even walking yet, but put it up anyway—why not?) and, again, anything else that occurs to you as a possible, however farfetched, emergency need.

Naturally if your baby has a special health problem, you'll alert her to that—but equally naturally, you're not likely to leave a sick infant in a stranger's hands unless there's some overriding urgency. If such a thing should happen, ask your doctor to recommend someone. The teen-ager next door might be perfectly adequate, but it's not a chance you'll want to take. This is a special situation, and it really can't be covered by these general rules.

AND MAKE HER PART CLEAR

Also in the information notebook—after you've talked them over with your candidate—are your specifications about what she may and may not do while she's working for you. Be thoughtful enough to remember that she's going to get hungry or maybe just want a snack, and either tell her she's free to help herself or show her where you'll leave something for her. To my knowledge, there's no way of getting her not to watch television—nor is there any reason, really, to think that just because she's got her eye on the tube, she won't have an ear out for the baby, not with this television-trained generation. But if she is going to watch, remind her to keep the sound down.

Would she like to bring along some favorite records? If your husband will allow it, show her *exactly* how to use your record player. If he won't stand for that, borrow a portable or tell her she may bring along her own. If she's going to browse among your books and magazines, gently suggest that she put them back when she's finished. I wouldn't do that the first time, by the way. That's the sort of thing you might do only if, after she's sat for you once or twice, you feel she has a tendency to forget to tidy things up but is otherwise the perfect treasure.

May she use the phone? Don't give a teen-ager *carte blanche*. Remind her that you will be checking in once during the evening (you should, but only once) to make sure things are fine and that you'll be concerned if you can't get through. You probably won't be concerned, really, since the favorite line of all parents who can't reach their homes because the line is busy is, "There's nothing to worry about because if someone's talking on the phone, they're alive, anyway." But she should be aware that, while she's working for you, the work, not her social life, comes first.

Teen-agers have absolutely no sense of time when they're hooked into one end of a phone. Tell her she may make, or receive, calls *in moderation* (don't say within reason, because her definition of reason is something very far from yours!) or—if you really mean it—tell her calls are off limits. But if you do, you may not get her again—perhaps none of her friends, either.

As far as the use of your home is concerned, if there's anything or any place that's off limits, tell her so. Perhaps you'd rather she didn't explore your bedroom or move anything on your husband's desk. Don't return to find that she has innocently mixed up some important letters he's working on to make room for her social studies research material. If she may use your typewriter, say so; if she wants to bring her own, show her where she can place it.

Give her coasters or paper napkins to prevent her from putting down, absentmindedly, a damp Coke glass on your best end table. Does she smoke? This isn't the time or place for missionary work; if you absolutely will not allow her to smoke around your baby or in your absence, she either doesn't smoke or she doesn't sit for you. If you don't feel that strongly about it, make sure she has plenty of ashtrays or the holes in your carpet will be—more or less—your own fault.

Now, visitors. This has to be your decision, made on the basis of your own ideas or the particular person who's sitting for you or a combination of both. I'd suggest that you tell a first-time sitter that you do not want her to have a visitor, and then add—according to your own principles— that it's because it's her first crack at your home and baby and you want everyone to get used to everything about it or that it's because you don't approve of visitors at any time when she's sitting and you simply don't allow your sitters that privilege. Tone it down any way you can, make it pleasant and acceptable, but if that's the way you feel, make it firm.

It's somewhat easier and more fair to tell her that she can't have visitors of either sex because if you tell a teenager she may have a girl friend visit but not a boy, she's going to say, "But why?" Then you'll be into something that really isn't your problem or, to be quite frank, your business —unless it's a young person you know very well, care about and want to get into a running debate with on all sorts of human problems that you won't have to take on with your own baby for another twelve years or so. You might want to do just that—get into a debate—because you can learn a lot that way; but at the moment it's not your prime concern.

With an older person, of course, the situation is entirely different. The question of a visitor probably won't come up. If it should, make your decision on the basis of the person you're dealing with. If your baby's going to be asleep, it might be very pleasant for your sitter to have a friend with whom to chat and share a cup of coffee.

YOUR PART OF THE BARGAIN

Baby-sitting is a two-way street. Having made it very clear what you expect of her, remember that she has a right to expect certain things of you as well. Unless you've made a definite arrangement about such little household chores as the still-dirty dinner dishes, don't leave them in the sink and rush off with a careless, "You won't mind doing those for me, dear, will you?" She will, and she should—unless, as I said, that's been your understanding from the first and you're prepared, if you think she feels it's over and above her baby-sitting duties, to pay a little extra for it. If you're willing and make it very clear, she'll probably do them gladly.

Which brings up the matter of money. Get this absolutely straight from the first. Know the going rate in your locality; expect to pay it or even do a little bit better for an outstanding sitter. Get it clear and businesslike before the first occasion arises. It's a business arrangement; treat it that way, and you'll be helping her to do so as well.

Even if you've met your baby-sitter in advance and she's seen your household setup and perhaps the baby has had a chance to get used to her (though that's a real extra and can't always be arranged), have her come in at least fifteen minutes ahead of time on the night she's going to sit. Certainly this is an absolute must the first time she comes. Get the baby—if he's awake—used to her presence. (Try to have him ready for the night, if not asleep, before she arrives.)

And never allow a sitter, as distinguished from a mother substitute, to bathe your baby. After she's come once or twice it's a good idea to let her feed him; that's about the best way for the two of them to get to know each other. (But the first time you won't want her responsible for picking him up and putting him down or even—unless she's practiced under your eye—for changing him.)

Review with her everything you told her the first time. Put the notebook out where she won't be able to forget that everything she'll need to know is there—first, of course, having added in big round letters all the information about where you'll be tonight and when you'll be home and how she can reach you—if possible—in the event that she decides it's necessary. Baby-sitters are human, too; they occasionally get upset stomachs. Or she might want to double-check about whether to give the baby orange juice or milk if he wakes up and seems to want something.

On the night when she's actually sitting, there's another kind of visitor problem you have to discuss with her. Are you expecting someone—a delivery, an out-of-town relative come to visit, *anyone* who might come to the door? By far the best thing is to make sure there will be no such event. Then, as you're not expecting anyone, tell her so clearly and add that she is not to admit anyone at all. Better to have an unexpected friend insulted than to take any chance of an unwelcome intruder while you're away from home.

THE UNFORESEEN

There are invariably problems that arise and that you have absolutely no way of anticipating. Usually they're trivial, though they can be annoying—and not the least is your annoyance with yourself for not having thought of the possibility. I have in mind an occasion a while ago when some young city-dwelling friends of mine managed to get a student nurse from a nearby hospital to baby-sit. She and their three-year-old already knew one another, she was a fine young person, and the parents went off without a care in the world, secure in their sitter's good sense and the reassuring sound of the chain lock being put on as she closed the apartment door behind them. The only trouble was that that chain was still in place when they got home. The nurse was asleep and they couldn't waken her. They finally had to call the police, who in turn called an all-night locksmith to get the door open.

"I'm kind of a heavy sleeper," the girl told them a little sheepishly. They couldn't help replying that, yes, they had noticed.

How could you protect yourself against that kind of mishap? They certainly didn't give up the sitter, who was wonderful in all respects. The next time they went out they suggested that if she felt sleepy, she was to lie down right inside the front door so that—just in case—they'd be able to poke her through the opening and get her up. But she never went to sleep on the job again.

There's another one of your responsibilities, by the way. When you've told your sitter about what time you'll be home, *be* home. If you're not sure, tell her that, too, and if she thinks she's going to fall asleep, have her lie down near the phone or in the same room with the baby so that she can (hopefully) hear him if he wakes. But it's better by far not to ask too much of her endurance.

Most youngsters tend to fall into the heavy kind of sleep that overcame our student nurse just mentioned. Get home when you said you would, or at least on the early side, and if you're going to be held up, telephone and alert the sitter. Then have her money ready—having figured out on your way home just how much it will be and being sure to turn any part of an hour that's hanging over into a full hour instead of paring it down to what ten extra minutes come to.

You won't "spoil" your sitter that way; she'll just decide you really are the greatest people to sit for and she wants to do the greatest sitting job she can for you in return. And then you make sure she gets home all right. Preferably, your husband walks or drives her home and waits until he's sure she's safely inside. That's another part of *your* job, whether your sitter is very junior or very senior.

THE DAYTIME SITTER

Any day now you may want someone to stand—or sit—in for you in the daytime. You won't do it when your baby's only a couple of weeks old, but in a little while you're going to have, or want, to get away "from all that" for a couple of hours even if it's only to go all by yourself to a movie or walk through a big, exciting store just to see what they're showing. Daytime sitting requires a little more of your sitter unless you have an infant—but the wise way to handle it is not to ask too much of her. Don't, for example, leave her with the responsibility of taking your baby for his outing; do it yourself before you go.

The best way to lay the groundwork is to have her come in—paying for her time, of course—and go through a couple of hours with you while you're doing your normal thing. That way she can see exactly how you handle your baby, how you talk to him, what his favorite toys are, what he means when he makes certain sounds, and where everything is—even though that's already written down in your information book, of course.

Like the information book, the rest of the rules are much the same as those I've outlined for your nighttime sitter. Any information she might possibly need must be thought out ahead of time and prepared for—by *you*. Show her how to change the baby, and have her do it more than once under your eye, being absolutely certain she understands that she's never to move away from him or take her hand off him, even for a split second.

If your baby's still on formula, have it ready and explain exactly how it is to be warmed and how the baby's accustomed to taking it—in what position you hold him—so that there won't be any two ways about that important procedure. Don't ask her to prepare the formula. And unless your baby is going to be napping the whole time she's there, don't ask her to take on any small household chore like vacuuming the living room rug—or any big chore, for that matter. Her job is your baby.

Before a sitter does more than that for you, she should be someone who's taken care of your baby several times, who knows her way around him and your home and whom you trust completely to do whatever is necessary and also to use her own judgment in case something comes up you haven't thought of. Once you've satisfied yourself that you have such a person, it's not really possible for you to learn from a book what you have to tell her. She'll know already what she previously didn't know and should ask about, or you'll instinctively be alert to any holes there might be in her preparation—or the two of you will be able to figure it out together.

THE MOTHER SUBSTITUTE

As I said at the start of this chapter, if you're going to be out of the house on a regular basis—probably working—then you need someone to take your place as the baby's mother. You might be lucky enough to have an ideal arrangement fall into your lap . . . a friend or relative who's really "your kind of person" and who's widowed or divorced or finds that with her own children at college or married, she's lonely and bored, or another young mother . . . we're dreaming, now, but after all some dreams *do* come true. Or perhaps you inherit a marvelous sitter, with long experience in being fully responsible for children, from a friend who no longer needs her. Otherwise, you ask around.

Don't be shy about discussing your problem with anyone who seems to have good sense and is willing to listen. The more people who know what you're looking for, the better your chances of coming across the person you need. Talking is a form of advertising, in this case, and I'd suggest that it's the only form you should go in for. Putting an ad in the newspaper, or answering one cold, is a risky business. You might be getting the most wonderful person in town, with a suitcase full of references that check out gloriously—but it's awfully hard to make a decision that involves the intimate, prolonged care of your baby on the basis of a few interviews and a few letters.

This is the kind of need that an agency could probably fill best. There are plenty of agencies that specialize in child-care help. Sometimes they call themselves by such names as Proxy Parents, or Stand-in Parents—something to indicate that they know they are being asked to provide more than just feeding and cleaning-up care. If you're planning to leave your baby while he's still under three months old, you might feel more secure if you can get a baby nurse.

She'll be trained and experienced enough for the physical care of any baby, and since she's doing the work, you have to assume or at least hope that she also loves babies—and more, that she's going to understand that you want yours treated with love and understanding, not just kept full and dry. You have to be careful and choosy, though; baby nurses sometimes elect this particular branch of activity because they only enjoy babies who are too small to offer anything more than physical problems. They may not like playing with a child who's beginning to sit up and notice the world and is maturing enough to show a little personality and perhaps a little disposition to fight back. Also, nurses are *expensive*.

So is a full-time housekeeper, of course—but we're assuming that you're going back to work precisely so that there will be extra money. (If you need full-time baby care for an illness or some other family emergency, that's not so pleasant—but don't let the tension make you forget that you still have to find the best, the most nearly right, person you can, and that the expense is just going to be one of those unfortunate extra pressures life puts on us from time to time. Don't take someone who'll "come for less" if you're not sure she's also better or at least as good; this is hardly the time to economize!)

Even an agency can't turn up the right person if you don't have a mind's-eye view of what you need. Don't try to work it out by phone. It's far better for you to go down to the agency's office and let an experienced interviewer size *you* up while you're telling her what you want. She'll have a better chance of matching you up with the applicants she has available. Don't conceal any of your requirements or even your personal quirks.

If the interviewer looks at you coldly and remarks, "You're quite particular, aren't you!" say yes indeed, you certainly are when it's a question of your baby's care and safety.

Now let's assume that the agency—or the kindly fates—have turned up someone for you who looks and sounds as though she were made to order. Hope—but take nothing for granted. The best way, indeed the only way, to find out if what is glittering before you really is pure gold is to make an arrangement to have your candidate come in and work with you while you're still at home, for—at the very least—a week. This is a very important decision you're making, and if it doesn't happen to be the right one, you'll unfortunately have to take time off from your work after a while in order to find and break in somebody else. It makes more sense to delay going into your own job until your replacement has worked into the one you want her to fill.

THE SITTER'S HEALTH

If you find your wonderful mother-substitute in an agency, it should be able to provide a health record on her to ease any worries you might have about such things as skin disorders that might be catching, TB or any other chronic health problems. But if you've solved your need through a personal recommendation, you'll have to check into your candidate's health on your own. If she herself offers the information, or a doctor's checkup report, wonderful—that shows experience plus the right sense of responsibility. But if you find that you're the one who has to bring it up, don't hesitate to do so.

9

Another Word for Love

At an amazingly early age, your baby will exhibit a mind and a personality all his own. Even a very young baby may, for example, protest against having a bath or being diapered, and you must gently but firmly overrule those protests.

In the weeks, months and years to come, there will be many, many instances in which you will have to employ gently firm discipline and provide guidelines and boundaries to keep your young one under control, for a small child simply does not have the experience and wisdom to judge what he should or should not do. For your child's protection, in many cases you must judge for him.

BE BABY'S FRIENDLY GUIDE

Some mothers make the mistake of believing that discipline involves a contest of wills, in which she has to "win" and the baby must "lose." That's not really what discipline is all about. Besides being the baby's mother, you are his guide and his friend, not his master. Discipline is another word for love, really—because you love your little one, you want to show him the right way, show him how to grow up to be the kind of person who can cope with the world around him, who can accept and deal with frustrations and setbacks and sorrow as well as with love and joy and pleasure.

On the other hand, it's a mistake to confuse love with permissiveness and to fear that your child won't love you if you don't give him his way all the time. Children really do sense the need for rules. They sense the need for knowing the limits beyond which they cannot go and they welcome your guidance, although, being human, they may make surface protest against it.

I remember that years ago I went with a friend to visit a young mother whose only child, a boy, was somewhere between four and five years old. This was at a time when excessive permissiveness was all the rage—psychologists solemnly taught that if you said no to a child, you would permanently damage his little ego; if you crossed him, kept him from doing anything he took into his head to do, you would injure his psyche and he would grow up psychologically crippled.

The little boy, Kevin, whose home we were visiting, had just been given a junior tool set—a saw, hammer and other tools, all of a size for small hands to cope with. As my friend and I chatted with the mother, Kevin brought in his tool chest, sat down on the floor and began to try to saw one leg off the coffee table. I called the mother's attention to it, thinking she was so wrapped up in our conversation she hadn't noticed.

"I know," she said. "But I daren't tell him not to. He's being exploratory, and that's good for him."

"It's not very good for the coffee table," my friend said a bit tartly.

"Well, the tools aren't sharp, of course. He won't be able to get the leg off."

True, he couldn't. But he could damage the finish badly —and he did.

A few moments later he moved over by my friend and started lunging at her leg with the saw. She reached down, caught his hand and said pleasantly, "No, Kevin. No! I'm not going to let you ruin my stockings."

"Oh, that's terrible," his mother cried. "You said *no* to him. You must never say no to a child!"

As you can imagine, we left shortly after that. Outside the house I said to my friend, "What do you suppose is going to become of that poor little boy?"

"He'll end up in reform school," my friend predicted.

Mothers have to learn to be neither too rigid nor too permissive. Each extreme is just that—too extreme. But between those extremes there's a wide leeway, leaving plenty of room for those who propose to discipline with love and common sense—and fortunately, that applies to most young mothers.

THE DIFFERENCE BETWEEN NEEDS AND WANTS

While your baby is under nine months of age, you'll be concerned mostly with fulfilling your child's needs—his needs for food, sleep, love, play. Sometime between that nine-month age and the time he's a year old, you'll begin to help him distinguish between needs and wants. But before that you've been laying the groundwork for discipline by being consistent. Baby learns to love you and to depend on you through the constancy and the consistency of your care for him. You feed him at regular intervals—but not on so rigid a schedule that you wake him up so he can get his next feeding on the dot of what you think is the "right" time, according to schedule. Neither do you feed him only when it suits your convenience and let him go hungry until you are good and ready.

The same is true of his bathing, his playtime with you as he gets a little older. You are constant and consistent and, even though baby doesn't reason this out, he senses that those are two good qualities, two that make his world a good and happy place to live in. You are there when he needs you. You love and comfort him. He learns to count on you for good things.

And so, when you begin to help him understand the difference between acceptable and unacceptable behavior, he is still counting on you for the good things and finds your discipline acceptable, too. Again, he doesn't reason it all out, but he senses: "If mommy says this is wrong, it must be wrong."

CONSTANCY AND CONSISTENCY

Constancy and consistency in you build trust in baby. Babies need certain restrictions because those restrictions build up trust. For example, your little one must be confined sometimes—by the sides of his crib, for example. He feels fenced in. He'd rather not have that fence between him and the world. But you keep those crib sides up for his own protection, and if all your behavior is constant and consistent, he will sense that there is a reason for the restraint.

Later on there will be many other restraints. Some of them you will have to exercise more quickly and more forcefully than you would like to for the best results, but they are necessary—for example, if a toddler is about to run into the road in front of a car, you'll grab him instead of simply saying quietly, "Let's go the other way now," and hoping for the best. The danger is too great for the calm exercise of "positive" discipline.

But if you've been consistent and constant in your behavior toward him, he will understand that you acted in his own best interests—even if he is frightened by your swift movement and, because you were afraid for him, by your raised voice. If he is frightened, you'll cuddle and comfort him and explain—even if you don't expect him to understand entirely—why you acted as you did.

Some mothers light upon a system of discipline that is a sort of "an eye for an eye" policy. If a toddler slaps someone, he is slapped back—not too hard, but enough to know that it hurts. If he pinches, he is pinched. If he bites, he is bitten. This may seem to work well for a time, but really, it's based on a false premise. In the first place, many children don't seem to be wounded by the sting of the slap—they take the whole thing as a big fun game. Even if they don't, the system is bound to break down.

A young mother I knew a number of years ago tried this system. For a while she swore by it. Then one day the older little girl threw her young sister's favorite stuffed dog into the fireplace, where a hot fire was burning. (She shouldn't have been allowed to get that close to the fire in the first place!) The mother went and got *her* favorite toy, a teddy bear, and threw it into the fire. That was cruel. Children's attachments to one particular toy are great and should be respected. By this time she had two bitterly weeping, broken-hearted little girls on her hands. A moment later, when the older child tried to push the younger one into the fire, the whole "eye for an eye" system collapsed.

THREATS ARE NO GOOD

Another system that breaks down is the one that depends on threats—particularly threats that can't or won't be carried out. One example of this is the child, older than a toddler but still too young for constant responsibility, who is given a pet and told that he must take care of him. He must give the dog his supper, for example, every afternoon at five. For a few days he constantly asks if it's five o'clock yet, so eager is he to feed his puppy. But then the novelty wears off and he forgets. He is reminded. He does his chore reluctantly.

One day, absorbed in playing a game with a little visitor, he refuses to feed the dog. He is too young to understand that with the pleasure of having the puppy goes the responsibility of caring for him. "All right," the mother says, "if you won't feed your dog I'll give him away." But she has made a threat she won't keep.

The whole family is by now attached to the dog. She really doesn't mind feeding him—it takes only a moment as she goes about the kitchen getting the family dinner ready. But she has made a serious mistake. She's taught her son that she doesn't always mean what she says. She's taught her son that he can go ahead and do as he likes and she may threaten but won't carry out the threat.

What should she have done—given the dog away? No, she should have refrained from making an idle threat in the first place. She should have thought it through. She should have asked herself: "If I say it, will I carry it out?" If the answer is no then she should not say it.

In fact, threats of any kind are at best ineffective and at worst seriously damaging to the relationship between mother and child. Statements of the factual consequences of an act are much more effective. "If you put your hand on the hot pot, you will be burned and it will hurt very much."

... "If you don't put on your sweater, you will be very cold outdoors." Pleas are inappropriate, too. "Oh, please put on your sweater—I'm afraid you'll catch cold." If the child is at the age where he is testing how much he can get away with, the answer will probably be *no*.

It's much better to start out on the other foot by saying, "It's chilly outdoors today. We'll both put on sweaters." If the answer is no, she has an alternative ready. She says, pleasantly but firmly, "Then we will not go outdoors." Not a threat, a statement—and she sticks to it. If, in a few minutes, the youngster says, "Let's go outdoors," she gets her sweater and his and matter-of-factly puts them on.

NEITHER TOO LITTLE NOR TOO MUCH

We were speaking a moment ago of needs and wants. It's up to you to help baby learn the difference—and to learn, too, that not only needs are gratified but sometimes reasonable wants, too. It's those that add spice and pleasure to life— most needs are simple, and life would be pretty dull if we had only our needs fulfilled and never, never got any of our wants. The needs, of course, you will take care of. The wants? Try to strike a happy balance. Sometimes your youngster will demand something that he wants, not needs. If the fulfilling will do him no harm, allowing him to have it will give both of you pleasure. But he has to learn that "I want it" isn't necessarily followed by his getting whatever it is. You, his mother, are in control.

Try to find the happy medium that exists between too much control and too little, between undercontrol and overcontrol. Undercontrol is the road to lost control. Overcontrol makes you a jailer as well as a mother. But always, always err on the side of being overgenerous with your affection. Children sometimes equate gratification of wants with love. If you must deny wants—and often you must, for the good of the child, whether it be his stomach or his personality —make sure, by open and constant expressions of your affection, that he understands that you love him anyway. He will learn that it is *because* you love him that you guide him, discipline him, sometimes deny him certain things.

When your child is between nine and twelve months old,

he will begin to respond to a variety of kinds of training. Remember, you are not primarily interested in getting your way. You are primarily interested in guiding him so that his way is the good way, so that he learns to understand the difference between the good and the bad way. To begin with, avoid problem situations as much as you can. If, for instance, you want to eat candy—and your figure allows you to do so without guilt—have your little treat while your toddler is taking his nap. That way you've avoided telling him he can't have any candy without being able to offer a reason that he will understand. (Did *you* understand "It's not good for you!" when you were his age?)

That's one guideline: *avoid the occasion of a problem if that is feasible.* A second: *distract his attention if you can.* Your aim in life is not to get into a fight with your toddler; if you can turn his attention to something other than the inappropriate want he is making known, fine. Of course, if he expresses the same inappropriate want many times, he'll soon learn not to be distracted—and that is just as well, because distracting repeatedly on the same account only postpones the want for him rather than letting him know it cannot be gratified.

Distraction works well in many instances. If, for example, you've taken him shopping and he demands a gaudy can of food you don't want, wheel him past, at the same time asking him if he will hold the nice, rattly box of cereal for you in your shopping cart.

A third guideline: *reward your child for appropriate behavior with your approval.* "With your approval"—those are the key words. Not with a treat, not with candy—with your approval. You and your husband are the most important people in your child's world—he wants and needs your approval. "What a good boy you are!" when he has done something you wanted him to do can mean a great deal to your youngster. Just as you won't make threats you won't or shouldn't keep, you won't make promises you can't or won't keep either, whether promises of reward for good behavior or any other promises. You want your child to have faith in you and in your ability to keep your word and your sincerity in wanting to keep your word.

A fourth guideline: *make clear your disapproval of unsuitable behavior*. Just as the child wants to win your approval, he dreads losing it. So you must be certain to make clear that it is his behavior you disapprove of, not the child himself. Instead of making a general statement such as, "You're a bad boy!", it is better to say, "You make Mommy angry when you don't put your toys away after you're through with them." That way you have pinpointed the specific reason for your disapproval and the child will understand that it is his behavior you dislike, not him.

DON'T CONFUSE YOUR YOUNGSTER

Sometimes it's possible to employ several of these guidelines at once or in sequence, but try to move slowly and with calm, so that your youngster will understand what you're getting at, without being confused by a number of different reactions on your part. Remember to show your love for him —and that's not hard, is it, because those little humans are so very lovable!—as you discipline him.

One of the traps mothers often fall into is telling some third person, in the youngster's presence, about some mischief he got into and making it clear, by laughter and tone of voice, that you really thought it was pretty cute. This will almost guarantee that he will repeat the behavior. Restrain yourself— at least until a time when there's no danger of the young one's overhearing you.

By the same token, try not to show a mixture of admiration and disapproval when your youngster has done something you really don't want him to do. He'll like the reaction, make up his own mind that "she really doesn't mean it" and repeat the behavior in order to elicit the same response. Make every attempt always to exhibit the same reaction to the same behavior. If you laugh and hug the child on one occasion and reprimand him on another for doing the same thing— perhaps because your temper is frazzled and your fuse consequently short the second time—you'll leave him hopelessly confused.

HOW ABOUT YOUR OWN SELF-DISCIPLINE?

In guiding the baby who is just beginning to learn the

limits that discipline will allow him to go, try to suit the action to the word. For example, some people clear the house of their valuable possessions so that breaking them won't be an occasion for trouble. (That's the first guideline—avoiding the occasion for a problem.) But you can't of course strip the house entirely. If baby reaches for something he can't have, don't simply say, "No, no." Give him another clue. Tap the reaching hand gently as you say no to him. Not slap—tap. Just let him know it is his hand that is getting him into a situation that will earn your disapproval.

Guidance requires discipline on your part, too. If, for example, you find that your toddler, while your back is turned, has pushed the kitchen chair over to the cupboard, has climbed up and is now standing, chortling happily, on the counter, what do you do? The thing you don't do is yell. In the first place, that might startle him so that he will fall. Or it might inject so much drama into the situation that he'll repeat it as soon as possible in order to hear you scream again.

So what do you do? Try walking across to him firmly, frowning as you do so, and say, "No, you must not climb up on the counter," lift him down and set him on the floor, put the chair back where it belongs and be disapprovingly aloof with him for a short time. A short time is all that is necessary—indeed, a longer time is unnecessarily cruel because he will have forgotten the reason for the trouble and decide that for some mysterious reason you don't like him.

Moderation is the watchword here—and it's the key to good discipline. A moderate course between strictness and permissiveness gets the best results because it teaches the child that there are boundaries to his behavior that he must respect and at the same time never allows him to feel deprived of your love and support. You must understand yourself and your own attitudes before you can hope to discipline a child well. And you must reach a meeting of minds with your husband on the subject of discipline too. If one of you is excessively permissive and the other excessively strict, the little one will at first never know what is expected of him. Later, he'll begin to play one of you off against the other in order to get his way.

Make a pact with your husband, too, that neither of you will interfere with any disciplinary measure of the other. Countermanding each other's orders, or even suggestions, will lead to chaos. Talk it over later, out of the child's hearing, and settle the point—but don't do it in front of the child. That, too, will quickly give him the idea that he can get mommy and daddy into such a disagreement that they'll forget all about the original cause and he can go on his way doing just as he pleases.

It's important to have the courage of your own convictions. Once you have made a rule, enforce it—don't back down. Don't say to yourself, "Oh, poor little fellow, he's only a baby—I'll let him do it this one time." This, again, leaves the child not knowing where he stands, not knowing what the boundaries are, if the boundaries are different on Thursday from what they were on Tuesday.

DON'T WORRY TOO MUCH

It's also important for you not to worry excessively over your attitude toward your child. When he's a newborn, you look down on him, lying in his bassinet, and think he's the sweetest child who ever drew the breath of life. It doesn't even cross your mind that he will sometimes make you very angry, that he'll sometimes do things that outrage you. Anger and outrage are human reactions and you are a human being. You won't be the only mother who's ever been cross with her child. If you were, this would be a world full of little angels—sweet, but dull!

A little anger sometimes, a bit of outrage once in a while, is quite normal. The reason most of us don't feel anger and outrage at our children more often is that we've developed a reasonable set of rules that all abide by most of the time. We've been constant and consistent in our discipline, and our children know what the rules are and what the boundaries are and respect them most of the time. The rules and boundaries keep them lovable—and loving.

Most children go through a stage where they feel that *no* is the right answer to every question. This is the stage where you'll learn to frame what you say so that it can't elicit a no response. Of course, this is impossible all the time, but you'll quickly learn not to create occasions for unacceptable behavior by asking questions to which the little one can gleefully tell you "No!" For instance, it's simpler, when your child is between one and three years old—the *no* years—to say, "Come and sit down—it's time for lunch," rather than "Would you like to sit down and eat your lunch now?"

It's also easier on both of you if you don't saddle a young child with too many choices. He finds making such choices very difficult. His inclination is to choose both or neither as a way of solving the problem. So avoid, "Would you like a peanut butter sandwich or a cheese sandwich?" Offer one or the other without comment. (On the other hand, if he volunteers, "I want a peanut butter sandwich," there's no reason in the world—except contrariness on your part—to give him cheese instead and expect him to eat it without protest.)

Normal children are basically "good"—when you teach them, by word and by example, what acceptable behavior is and if you are consistent and constant in expecting acceptable behavior. They want to behave acceptably, and do, most of the time.

A number of mothers have written me asking how they can teach their children to be polite—to say "please" and "thank you" and react with courtesy when the occasion calls for it. Of course, when he's old enough to understand, you can explain to a child why politeness is desirable—a simply worded explanation that good manners provide the oil that keeps the wheels of everyday living running a bit more smoothly.

However, long before his reasoning powers can accept such an explanation, he can begin learning from his parents and others around him. In a household where "please" and "thank you" and the other small courtesies are the usual and not the unusual thing, your little one will learn them and their use, just as he learns other words and their use from those around him.

EARLY THUMB-SUCKING IS NORMAL

Another problem many mothers write to me about is thumb-sucking—or, at least, they consider it a problem. They feel they're doing something wrong (or neglecting to do something right) that must be the cause of the toddler's sucking his thumb because they've read or heard that he does this to comfort himself. If he needs comfort, then something must be wrong.

Not necessarily. Up until the baby is six months old, most authorities agree, thumb-sucking is just another manifestation of the sucking reflex with which all babies are born, so that when they come into the world, they can take nourishment.

At about six months, most babies begin to assert their independence. They don't always want to be cuddled, for example. Sometimes, sitting on mother's lap, they'll sit up straight instead of relaxing into the circle of her arm. Or they'll push away the hand that's feeding them. They are trying their wings now. They don't want to be totally dependent. But when they're tired or out of sorts, they automatically revert to the time when they were totally dependent, when everything was done for them, when they didn't have to "think for themselves." Sucking was part of that early babyhood, and to comfort themselves they suck the handiest object—usually their thumbs.

Almost all babies suck their thumbs—some much more often than others—between the ages of three and seven months. Many suck their thumbs much longer—deriving comfort from it when they are tired or frustrated. Instead of a thumb, some babies suck on a pacifier. For a long while pacifiers were in disfavor, but now some doctors approve of the comfort they give a child. Whether your youngster sucks his thumb or a pacifier, it's really nothing to worry about. One impatient young mother wrote me concerning her eighteen-month-old youngster, "I used to think it was cute. But now he's beginning to look stupid with his thumb in his mouth!" No, he doesn't look stupid—he looks like a baby, and he *is* still a baby. Perhaps this mother should ask herself some questions: "Am I pushing him along too fast? Am I expecting—perhaps demanding—too much of him? Do I subconsciously want him to behave in a manner older than his actual age?"

Many devices to keep a young one from sucking his

thumb have been employed—and none of them works. There are nasty-tasting liquids with which parents paint the (what they consider to be) offending thumb. Sometimes the thumb is bandaged or covered with adhesive tape. Sometimes a cuff of cardboard or some other stiff material is placed around the elbow so that the arm can't be bent sufficiently to get the thumb up to the mouth. All these devices, and any others for the same purpose, are cruel. If you can't bring yourself to think of anything you consider to be for baby's own good to be cruel, think of it as useless—so what's the point? None works.

The baby becomes accustomed to the nasty taste and sucks his thumb anyway. Or he sucks the bandage, adhesive tape and all. With a cuff on his arm, he uses the other thumb; with a cuff on each arm he waits—frustrated and fretful and terribly unhappy—until the cuffs come off and he can start sucking again.

So don't bother—and don't worry. Very few babies will continue to suck their thumbs long past their first birthdays. Even if yours does, treat it as part of the growing-up process and don't try to break baby of the habit.

Some children who don't suck their thumbs—and even some who do—develop a passionate attachment to some other form of "comforter." It may be the corner of a blanket or a quilt or one particular diaper that, to you, seems no different from all the other diapers or a soft and cuddly toy or just a scrap of cloth that the baby has come by accidentally.

A toddler may want to carry this object of his affection everywhere with him. Such objects get increasingly dingy the more they are handled, but baby will protest violently if mother "borrows" it long enough to give it a good scrubbing. If by some mischance the object is lost or even temporarily mislaid—left by accident at grandmother's, for example—baby will be heartbroken. He may not be able to go to sleep until hours after his usual bedtime, finally dropping off to sleep from the sheer exhaustion of crying for the missing object.

It's usually impossible to break a child's attachment to such an object—and it's unnecessarily unkind to try. If you must wash it—and you'll certainly feel you have to after a while—take it away after baby is sound asleep, wash and dry it and have it ready for him when he wakes up. It's better to wash it before it gets very dirty—that way, its taste and smell won't be too much changed from the way the baby remembers it before he went to sleep.

COMFORT FROM CLINGING TO OBJECTS

This clinging to an object of comfort may last longer than thumb-sucking or it may be combined with thumb-sucking. But there's no harm in it, and if the child derives solace from the object, why try to break the habit? Sometimes it's possible to confine the problem somewhat—insist that the object be used only in the baby's room or inside the house—but often this won't work. So simply try not to be too upset by it. Your young one will probably outgrow his attachment by the time he's two or three years old. Meanwhile, when he's old enough to understand, drop a hint once in a while—something like, "You're getting to be a big, grown-up boy now, and pretty soon you won't need that old thing anymore, will you?"

A related problem is that of rhythmic movements a child makes; bouncing, jouncing and—much more frightening—head banging. Probably, some authorities say, he's learning rhythm—you'll find that these rhythmic movements often occur at about the same time baby becomes actively conscious of music heard on the radio or record player and tries to move in time to it.

If his bouncing and jouncing, particularly in his crib, become bothersome, as they can when he bangs the crib against the wall or jounces so that he moves it across the room, put a "bumper" of soft material between crib and wall and/or chocks beneath the front wheels of the crib so he'll be unable to move it. As for head banging, be sure everything he can bang his head against is something that is comfortably padded, and then stop worrying. He won't, as some mothers fear, "beat his brains out." And fortunately these actions are usually of short duration and most often occur when he's worn out and sleepy and confined to his crib.

One of the worries that mothers—especially mothers of first babies—have to cope with is the baby's setting up howls of protest the moment mom disappears from his sight. It's a real problem because, of course, you can't stay with him all the time. And anyway you shouldn't because he has to learn to be by himself. What to do? Well, you might try playing peekaboo with him around the door. Or, as you leave to go into the next room, tell him, "I'll be back," and when you return, "See, I came back." He won't understand at first, but soon he'll be able to associate the words with the actions. He'll understand that people do go away, but not for good.

It's not wise, however, to sneak out or to lie to him. His sense of security can suffer quite a blow from such actions. When you leave the house—leaving him in someone else's care, of course—your "I'll be back" will comfort him if he has already learned that you always do come back. It's a good idea to get a baby used, from infancy, to being left in the care of others for short periods. (It's good for you, too—you'll come back from your shopping trip or your movie with a friend feeling refreshed and much more able to take on again the demanding business of raising a baby.) And even if you are anxious about leaving baby, don't let him know it, ever. Say a cheerful, confident "Good-bye—I'll be back," and go!

TOILET TRAINING

Toilet training—how many mothers have agonized over it and how many more will agonize over it in the years to come! When is the best time to start? How should you go about training the toddler? Will you create tensions or antagonism in the child if you start too soon? Is it best to postpone training until the child can literally teach himself?

There's little point in trying to train a child who is too young to understand what you're trying to get at and isn't capable of the control necessary for him to respond to training. But once he does have the necessary understanding and control, you can begin to guide him in the right direction.

Many children have the first bowel movement of the day five to ten minutes after breakfast—if yours is one of those, you'll start by putting him on the "junior" toilet seat or on his own potty chair at the appropriate time, praise him and tell him what a big boy he's getting to be when you get the desired

No closer bond exists than that between a mother and her baby. Relax and enjoy those precious early months. *See pages 117–118.*

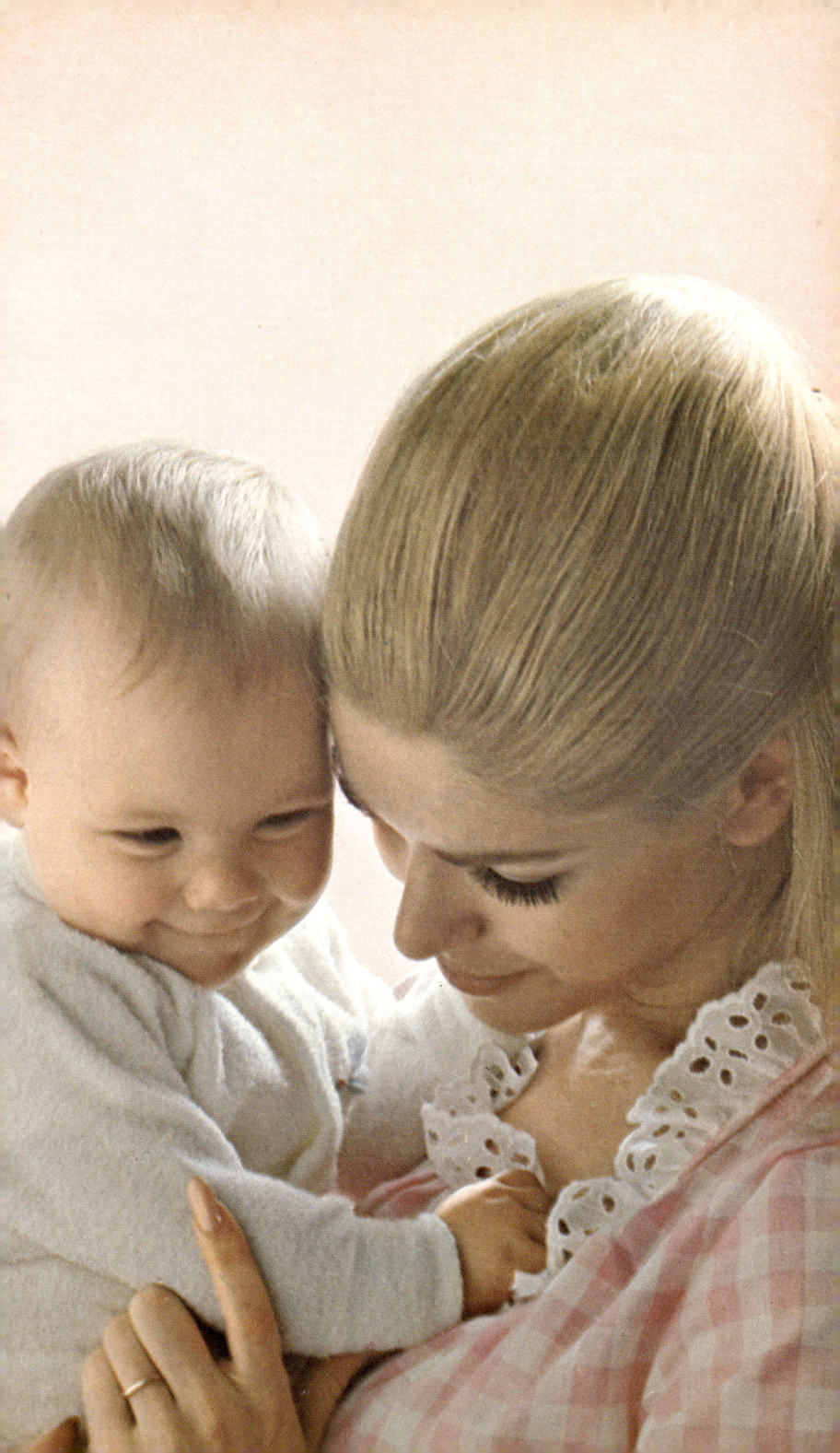

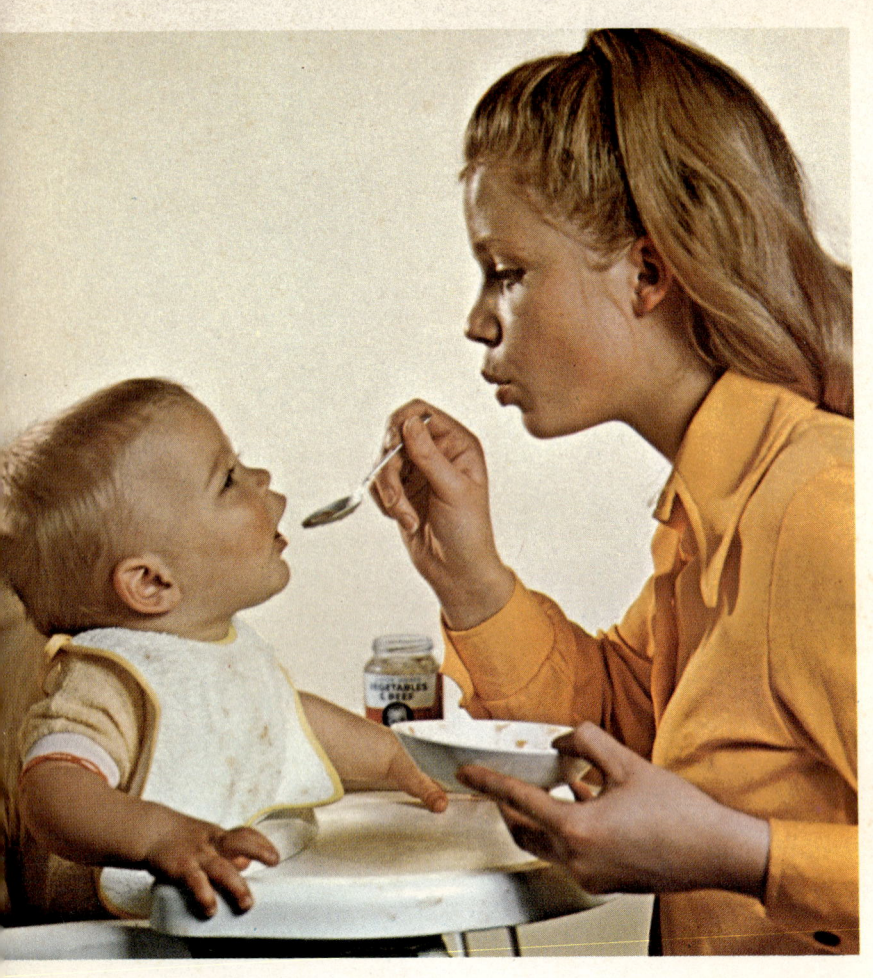

Great empathy can be established between your baby and his baby-sitter if the sitter feeds him. *See pages 98–113 for baby-sitting tips.*

The tenderness of little brother toward the baby can be touching. *See pages 131–132 for ideas on preparing a child for the new arrival.*

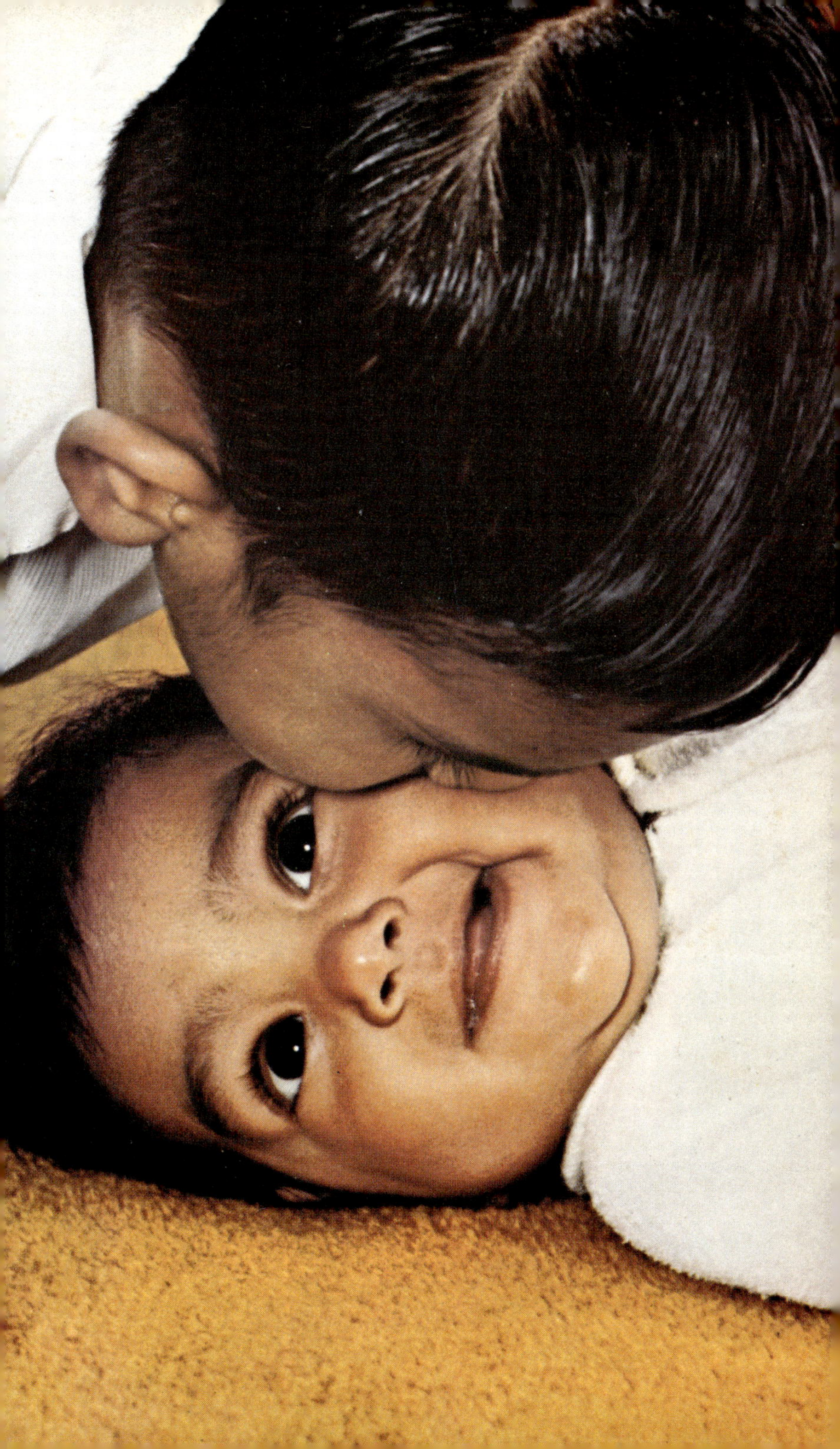

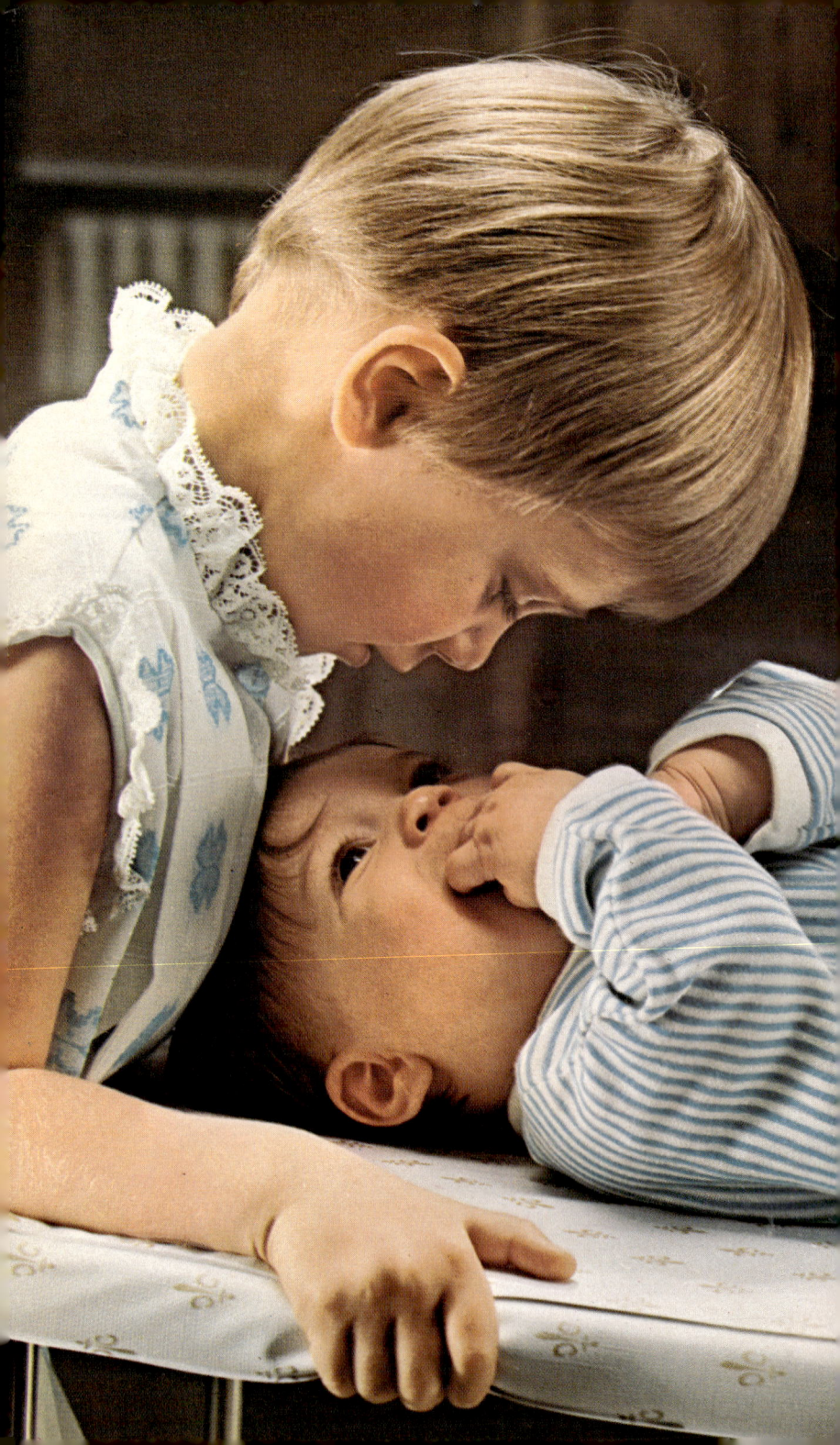

result. Even if your child is not yet this regular, you will soon learn the sign he makes before a bowel movement—a word, an expression on his face—and you can take him to the potty and praise him for a successful performance.

Five to ten minutes is quite long enough to keep him on the chair if you get no results. And be casual—don't act excessively disappointed. He'll soon get the idea. And expect setbacks, for there are bound to be some. Few, if any, children have ever been trained from the start without setbacks and accidents. You'll have to have patience, and it's important to be friendly and casual, important not to act as if the whole day turned on this event. Accidents are most likely to occur in exciting situations, such as when you're visiting another home, when traveling or simply when the youngster is playing out of doors and doesn't want to take time out from his play to go inside the house to the bathroom.

Above all, don't let toilet training turn you into a nag—all you'll do is develop antagonism between yourself and your child. In any form of teaching, you'll find that you will meet with far greater success if you encourage your child and praise him when he does what is wanted than you will by nagging and scolding him if he fails.

THOSE TERRIBLE TEMPER TANTRUMS

Temper tantrums, my mail tells me, have frightened more mothers than almost any other of the manifestations of growing up. These tantrums usually begin somewhere between the time the toddler is twelve to fifteen months old and rarely continue after he's three. They are usually caused by the fact that he wants to do something he has not the strength or stamina to do or to continue doing something long past the point where he's too tired to go on or, less often, because he wants something that for some reason he cannot have or he is overstimulated. You can help most by eliminating as many occasions as possible for such tantrums. Regulate his life wisely so that he doesn't get overtired.

Arrange your home so that there are not many things in his sight that he cannot have. Make sure he gets plenty of rest, that he's fed when he's hungry. Help him with his play or play with him so that he doesn't get frustrated trying

Little sister will want to "mother" the baby—find things she can do so that she will feel part of the warm circle. *See pages 131–132.*

to accomplish something he can't hope to accomplish. You're the wise one—you have to be his guide and friend.

But with all the tactful regulation in the world, many children still have temper tantrums and some have them often. The tantrum usually starts with a cry of irritation and passes to the point where the child throws himself down on the floor, screaming and flailing about. Sometimes he will hold his breath—the thing his mother dreads most—even to the point of turning blue and passing out. (Don't be afraid of this. When he loses consciousness, he automatically will catch his breath and, usually, when he regains consciousness— a matter of thirty to forty seconds that can seem like as many years—the tantrum will be over.)

Above all you must learn to control yourself even if he can't control himself. The more you show him that you are frightened, the sooner he may get the idea that a temper tantrum is the ideal way to control mom. It may calm him if he is ignored; perhaps you can steel yourself and walk away from him, in case he is enjoying an audience for his display. But he may not be attempting to influence you—he may just have come to the point where he can't stand things the way they are one second longer. The business of growing up brings with it numerous infuriating frustrations.

Try distraction—and when distraction fails, as quite often it will, ignore the sound and fury, or try to. Don't bribe him —that's worse for him than it is for you, and bribing isn't dignified for a full-grown woman. Don't threaten him, either. It will do no good and make you feel foolish or unfeeling. And it won't help to try to reason with him—he's way beyond sweet reasonableness by now. Just let the tantrum run its course, and when it's over let him know you love him. Don't give in to him, though—that way lies infant blackmail, as he'll be quick to realize.

FRUSTRATION—A PART OF LIFE

If possible, you'll avoid tantrum-causing situations, of course. But don't make the mistake of trying to spare him all frustrating experiences. Life itself can be filled with frustrations, and he learns and develops by dealing with frustrations. Perhaps the tantrum develops because he's having trouble learning to put on his shoes. Don't take them away from him and put them on him yourself. That simply bypasses the frustration. He'll have to wear shoes all his life, so it's your business to help him learn how to put them on. How proud he'll be when he has mastered the technique!

Once again, try to be consistent in what you allow your child to do and what you don't allow him to do. If you let him have something dear to you to play with and later realize it wasn't a good idea and you deny the object the next time he asks for it, you're setting up an occasion for a tantrum. For you to be indulgent one day and strict the next creates uncertainty in the child—as it would in an adult in the same situation.

You will, of course, give your child a great deal of your attention, but there will be times when he'll have to wait his turn. Some children can't stand to have their mother talk on the phone and demand attention and create a rumpus whenever she does so.

One bright young mother I know came up with an excellent solution to this problem. She filled an old handbag—and you know how interesting handbags are to little ones!—with small items, old jewelry, a nonworking watch, a set of measuring spoons, a zipper, a bunch of buttons strung on stout thread. She keeps this "treasure bag" in a drawer near the telephone. Now, when she's on the phone, she gives her toddler the bag which keeps her gloriously occupied while her mother finishes her conversation in peace. It serves another purpose, too, this mother tells me; it keeps the youngster from wandering off and getting into mischief in another room, out of mother's sight.

Quite often when a youngster reaches the toddler stage, his mother will have another baby. How do you best prepare your first child for the advent of the second?

To begin with, *do* prepare him. Don't just "let things happen." If you don't tell him in advance, your absence from home and subsequent return with the new brother or sister will come as a terrible, distressing shock to the first child. Make a story of it: how you will be going to the hospital to get a new brother or sister, how grandma will come to take care of him and daddy while you are away, how he can help you care for the new baby when you bring it home.

Let the first child share in the plans for the new arrival. Consult him as you fix the bassinet, as you get the bathinette out of attic or storeroom and give it a coat of paint. (Don't fall into the trap of asking his direct advice, such as "What color shall we paint the chest of drawers for the new baby?" The answer is likely to be "Red!" And then you are faced with going along with the suggestion or talking him out of it. Say, instead, "Will you help me get the chest of drawers ready for the new baby?")

When you bring the baby home, suggests one smart mother, you might show the older child off to him, telling the baby that this is his wonderful big brother and about all the things that big brother can do that the baby is too little to do for a long time yet. It'll be a great help, too, if the people who come to see the new baby will make a big fuss over the older child first, so that he doesn't feel left out. Perhaps the older one can take the visitors in and show them the new baby, so he'll feel that he's part of the excitement. It's only natural that he should feel somewhat jealous, but if you make him feel important, make it clear that he's the "big boy" of the family, it will ease the situation a great deal.

You might also ask the older child's advice whenever you can, as you tend the new baby. "Which sweater shall we put on baby this morning?" or "Which toy shall we give baby to play with?" If your older child is a little girl, one young mother tells me, it works wonders to have her bathe, dress and feed her doll, accompanied by a little woman-to-woman conversation, while you are doing the same thing for the baby. It occupies her and it makes her feel that she's grown up and that she is taking part—it's even good early training for her future role as a wife and mother.

Studies show that little girls talk to their dolls in exactly the same way that their mothers talk to them. (Listen sometimes, as a way of checking up on yourself. Perhaps you'll hear that you are being a bit too strict or a little overindulgent!) The studies further tell us that years later, when the youngsters are grown up and have children of their own, they will be talking to their babies the same way they did to their dolls. Interesting to think about it, isn't it?

10

Play's the Thing

From the time that baby is an infant his play is much more than merely fun—it is absorbing, fascinating practice for his future life. Playing with his fingers and toes, for example, is exercise in becoming familiar with his "working parts" and in developing his coordination. Of course he's having fun while he's doing it—what absorbing, difficult project isn't thoroughly enjoyable as you surmount the obstacles to become highly skilled? Babies find this just as true as adults do.

By the time your little one enters first grade, he will have made a good start on his education. He will probably learn more in those years than he ever will again in any six-year span of his life. For instance: from a helpless newborn, unable to understand anything of the world about him, he will have changed into an independent person with a vocabulary somewhere in the neighborhood of 4,000 words in the English language, which is one of the most difficult languages in the world to learn. And in all that time, you will have been your baby's teacher!

Just the same, it's not wise to think of yourself in those

terms because if you do, you may lean too heavily on the teaching aspects of play, unwilling to devote time to what you may come to think of as "silly" play. Babies love nonsense, and play should be full of joyful spontaneity. Do what's fun—the education will rise out of the fun, not the fun out of the education.

LEARNING CAN BE FUN

Even if you aren't aware of it, your house is full of what teachers like to call "instructional materials." What are they? Books, magazines, newspapers, television, radio. There are certainly a measuring cup and measuring spoons in your kitchen. Perhaps there's a thermometer outside your window. There are labels on most of the food supplies you buy, and —doesn't everyone?—you'll have bills. What else? House plants or window boxes or perhaps a garden plot in the yard. You'll be cooking—measuring, beating, stirring, baking, boiling, broiling. There are birds in the trees outside—if you have a feeder, you can attract them to your window.

Squirrels scamper in the yard. Perhaps the dog next door will have puppies or the cat upstairs kittens. There are trees and shrubs outdoors. A visit to a farm will give a look at other animals—cows, horses, sheep, pigs. A visit to the supermarket with mommy teaches baby where and how we get the things we eat and use around the house. Every day will bring more lessons in the biggest job anyone will ever have: learning how life is lived. He will be learning to have a healthy, balanced personality; to get along effectively with others; to think critically; to work creatively.

That's a very impressive list, isn't it? And how will he learn all this? By living with his mother and father, by playing with his mother and father, by observing his mother and father. What a job for a little newborn, lying there in his crib! Don't worry, he'll manage it all very effectively and neatly, with your help, without ever being conscious of the learning process at all.

When the baby is brand-new, he hasn't much time for playing—eating and sleeping take up the major part of his days and nights. But all the time he's awake, you're really playing with him in a quiet way—you talk to him as you change his diaper, as you dress him, as you bathe him, as you cuddle him and as you feed him and bubble him, chuckle him under his chubby little chin in the hope of eliciting one of those wonderful love-everybody smiles that only babies have to offer. There's something so completely engaging about a baby that no one ever need fear he won't get enough attention. Even the most dignified and unsociable adults are inclined to break into grins and kitchy-koos at the sight of a baby.

As he gets a little older, you'll buy him or make him a simple "baby gym"—a string of objects of various shapes, some of them making various sounds, which you fasten across his bassinet, just within reach, to entertain him. And perhaps a mobile of bird or fish or butterfly shapes (you can easily make one) fastened to the foot of his crib or somewhere else in the room where he can watch the movement of its shapes and shadows. Or perhaps a balloon or two in bright colors, fastened well out of baby's reach—anything that will give him something to watch and that will, incidentally, help him to exercise and develop his eye muscles in the pleasantest possible way.

Pretty soon you'll start playing peekaboo with him, teaching him to patty-cake, counting his fingers and toes, fondly saying, "Where is baby's nose? *There* is baby's nose. Where are baby's ears?" He'll chortle with glee—and he'll be beginning to learn the names of the parts of his body.

BUILT-IN CREATIVITY

The toys you choose for your child need not be elaborate or expensive. In fact, as your child reaches an age to choose his own playthings, you'll be surprised at what he selects. Often a homemade rag doll is chosen over a costly stuffed toy that someone has brought him as a gift. Often improvised items will intrigue him more than those bought ready-made. Many toddlers' favorite objects are a pot with its lid, a set of nesting, graduated-sized measuring cups, measuring spoons on a ring and a big spoon. With such equipment a little one will amuse himself playing put-together, put-in and take-out, put-the-hat-on, and stir, stir, stir! You'll find that your child has built-in creativity and born-in imagination and is perfectly willing to exercise them. Be content to let him do so.

Books? You'll buy him some, and he'll receive others as gifts. But his favorite may be the one made by stringing brightly colored greeting cards together—Christmas yields a bonanza of such cards, as do other holidays and birthdays. By using *your* imagination and creativity, you can help your family budget while helping your child's development.

As your baby gets a bit older and begins to have periods of wakefulness longer than the time required to tuck away his nourishment, you'll probably devote a part of each wakeful period to playing with him. You'll find it wise, as these periods grow longer, to schedule playing with him toward the end of the time rather than when he first wakes up. Otherwise he'll expect the play to extend throughout his wakeful period and, of course, you will have other things to do. You can be companionable with him, though, whatever you're doing. Don't leave him in his bed, all alone. When you get him up, change him, feed him if it's feeding time, and then put him someplace that will allow him to watch you—playpen, baby seat, walker, jouncy baby chair—and so that you can talk to him.

THAT FRIENDLY LITTLE PAT

I once asked a very wise old woman, who was much in demand as a baby-sitter, the secret of her success with children. She thought about it a moment and said, "Well, I think it's because I never pass by a child, any child, without saying hello to him and giving him a little pat."

Your baby, sitting or lying and watching you as you go about your work, will soon learn to expect and appreciate that kind of companionable give-and-take with you. You'll find that he'll make a sound of pleasure as you come near, that his little hand will come up to pat you, too. You don't have to hold him on your lap all the time for you to enjoy him and for him to enjoy you. In fact, if you do, he may become too dependent on you, feeling that your lap is the only "right" place for him to be when he is awake.

TOYS AND THE PLAYPEN

When can you start using a playpen? Sooner than you

think—as a matter of fact, it's wise for the baby to become accustomed to the playpen before he's able to move about in it very much, at three or at the most four months. That will be before he's learned to sit up and crawl and before you've given him the additional freedom of being loose on the floor. If you get him used to the playpen at three or four months, when he's a bit older he won't consider it a prison. By the time he can sit up and crawl around a bit, he'll have fun trying to get to the various toys you'll put into his playpen.

When he reaches the creeping stage, put him in the playpen first, while you go about your work—be sure it's where he can see you, though—and then let him creep a bit at the end of his period of wakefulness before you put him down for his next nap or to bed for the night.

Those treasured stuffed dolls and animals that he so delights in "chasing" around his playpen can get pretty grimy —and the most-loved ones get the dirtiest. Your baby won't accept any substitute for his favorites, yet you don't want him playing with anything so disreputable. Clean the toys he likes best regularly, suiting the kind of cleaning to the toy itself, before they get to the point of no return.

Various mothers have given me some excellent tips on cleaning toys. One says she rubs dry cornstarch on fuzzy stuffed toys, lets them stand for a few minutes, then brushes the cornstarch out, leaving the toys nice and clean. Another says she uses cornmeal the same way, especially on furlike stuffed animals, and if the toys are very dirty, she tells me, heating the cornmeal quite hot—do it in the oven—works wonders. Another young mother tells me that she uses a commercial-type furniture upholstery cleaner on such toys— she says it even makes the toys' matted hair stand up again.

Yet another says she tosses the toys into the automatic washer with good results but warns against putting toys with plastic faces into the dryer—the dryer's heat, she says, makes the faces come out looking like well-chewed gum! She advises, instead, that you hang the plastic-faced toys out in the sun or in a warm place in the house and then, when they are dry, brush them to fluff up the surface.

Although a few authorities are against playpens, most of them agree that they are a fine solution to what can be a problem—how to keep the baby confined but still near you. If you set up his playpen in the living room or kitchen or wherever you will be, he'll enjoy watching and "talking" to you. When he reaches an age where he begins to pull himself to his feet, the playpen's railing offers sturdy support and its floor something substantial under his feet.

When he begins to "travel"—inch his way in small steps, holding on to something—the playpen offers a safe place for him to practice this new accomplishment of his. When the weather is pleasant, he can be in his playpen on the porch or out in the yard where you can keep an eye on him without having to hold him. Playpens can go with you on visits, too—they are particularly useful when you're in homes that are not babyproofed as yours is.

MAGIC AND IMAGINATION

The day will eventually come, though, when your youngster will not be content just to stay in his playpen with his toys and his stuffed companions. What will you do, since he must stay there at times, such as when you are cooking? Young mothers have shared with me some wonderful tips for making playpens more interesting. Here are some of them:

* Most babies are fascinated by mirrors and by playing with their own reflections. If you securely fasten an old-fashioned triple mirror outside the playpen, your young one will be charmed for ages, while you go on about your work. Imagine having not one, but three babies looking back at you, doing every single thing you do! Magic!

* If you place a number of toys in a large paper bag, your baby can have a grand time pulling them out, examining them, stuffing them back in again. If you keep two or three such treasure bags, you can alternate bags, and baby's playtime will be just one great surprise after another, with "new" playthings each day. Incidentally, this is one of those cases where improvised toys are as good or better than the fancy ones. Babies simply love an old key ring with its dangling keys, small empty boxes, empty plastic bottles and the like.

* If baby is watching you "playing" with your pots and pans, he'll like doing the same. A covered saucepan—perhaps with a Gerber Teething Biscuit inside for a surprise—can be a real treat.

* A detachable plastic basket, such as the ones that come with most strollers, is fine to hang on the inside of a playpen. Fill it up with his toys and your youngster will have a great time emptying it and filling it up again. (And also throwing the things outside the playpen so that they have to be retrieved by mommy—but that's part of the fun.)

Whether bought or made at home, simple toys are the best toys. Too-complicated playthings that frustrate the baby aren't any fun for him. Watch him—you'll see what he chooses to play with at every stage of his growth. It's almost always something simple. (Of course what's simple for six months is too simple, quite often, for the one-year-old.)

This isn't, authorities tell us, because little ones' minds are so simple—it's because they have such vivid, splendid imaginations that they can turn almost anything into a dozen other things! For example, your husband may have very much enjoyed his toy trains when he was a boy—but chances are he's forgotten at what age he played with them. He may want to buy his son a set of elaborate trains, electric or wind-up, that run on a track, as early as the baby's first Christmas.

But baby won't understand until he's several years old how to make such a set of trains operate. He won't be able to wind up the engine. He won't be able to hitch the cars to the engine and to each other. He won't be able to keep the whole works on the track—he'll give it a shove and over it will go.

Your husband will have a grand time with such a toy, but for the baby a much more simple one will be infinitely preferable. If you want to buy one, buy the kind made of a line of flat wooden blocks that link together very simply and easily. The locomotion is provided by a string attached to one of the blocks so that baby can pull it. He can use the blocks strung together or apart, he can pile them high—they can be a train, a number of boats, a truck with a trailer—

almost anything his imagination tells him that they are.

Or make such a toy for him by stringing together a number of empty boxes of wood or cardboard—empty cereal boxes will make a fine train. Add a round oatmeal or cornmeal box for variety's sake and perhaps a couple of smaller boxes that can "ride" on top of or inside the bigger ones.

THE SECRET OF BLOCKS

Blocks are something that almost all young children are delighted by. You can buy big bags of a number of varicolored wooden blocks of many shapes and sizes, some of them hollow, some solid. At first baby will just tumble these together, delighted by their movement. One day he will discover a great secret: blocks can be piled one on top of another. Indeed, several can be piled up to make a tower which eventually will come crashing down. Then he'll build another to topple over on purpose. Later, as he gets a bit older, the blocks can be laid out as the streets of a town, the buildings of a shopping center, other places that his widening knowledge of the world stimulates him to imagine the blocks to be.

Again, empty boxes can be his blocks—empty boxes of various shapes and sizes that he can pile up or lay out. He won't know the difference. He'll love them just as much as little Johnny Jones down the street loves his expensive blocks from the toy store.

An empty cardboard carton is another delight. Children love to "put themselves away," and yours will pretend the carton is by turns a bed, a house, a truck, a dozen other things. And perhaps, if you're lucky, he'll pack away his other toys in it at the end of a long, exciting period of play!

Another toy that can serve this double purpose is a toddler's wagon. He'll love pulling it after him—and he'll love loading it up with his other playthings. It can do doubleduty as a storage bin between playtimes. Here's a chance to teach your youngster neatness by making a game of picking up his toys and putting them away in his wagon "to wait for you" when his period of play is over. As long as he's constantly learning, as long as he's constantly developing new habits, it won't hurt him to learn the habit of neatness instead of just drifting into the habit of sloppiness and carelessness.

Of course, you won't be constantly nagging him to pick up his toys—that will spoil the fun and make him resent the toys themselves. And you won't refuse ever to let him mess up his room or another room by scattering things around—youngsters revel in that sort of disorder. But you can make a game of it by cheerfully assisting him to straighten things up when playtime is over.

When they are two years old or a bit more, little ones turn into copycats. Girls want to sweep and cook and wash dishes. Little boys want to shave and mow lawns and "fix" things. And both of them want to drive cars. Implements that mom and dad usually handle but that are on a scale small enough for little hands to cope with interest them then—toy brooms and sets of dishes and pots and pans and ironing boards and irons, toy lawn mowers and rakes and shovels and tools of various kinds. When little girls get a bit older, they want dolls and doll furniture, little boys trucks and cars.

LISTENING IS IMPORTANT

Part of the youngster's learning-play consists in listening to you talk to him about everything that the two of you are doing. Talk about anything and everything—you'll find it helps him learn. This is probably why an only child or the first child in the family tends to be more creative—he receives more adult attention than it's possible to shower on younger brothers and sisters. But be as constructive as you can in your talking.

For example, don't just put his sweater on him or even just say, "Let's put on your sweater." You'll be giving him more fun—teaching him more because all his learning is fun now—by saying, "Let's put on your blue-and-white striped sweater with the blue buttons," or "Now we'll put on your red coveralls with the puppy on the pocket." In giving him a cookie or a biscuit, say, "Here's a round cookie for you," or "Here's a square cookie."

When you go out on walks, call his attention to everything to be seen. "There's a squirrel—see his big, bushy tail?" And not just, "See the birdie?" but, "There's a robin—see his pretty red breast?" "There's a green house." "We're going into the meat market." "Would you like to hold mommy's brown gloves?" This kind of specific chatter will make life more interesting and rewarding for you and your child.

You'll find yourself inventing games to keep your young one amused while you get on with your household chores. One mother I know of keeps her youngster happy and occupied when she cleans out the refrigerator by letting him play what they both call "The Ice Game." She puts plenty of newspapers down under his little table and a good padding of bath towels on top of the table. Then she gives him an ice-cube tray with several ice cubes and an assortment of kitchen utensils, such as a big spoon, a funnel, a tea strainer, an old coffeepot, a plastic cup.

As she goes about her business with the refrigerator, her little one is busy popping ice cubes in and out of the various utensils and watching the "mysterious" way the ice cubes drip away and eventually disappear. She swears that since she invented the game, she finishes her refrigerator cleaning in record time.

CRAYONS, COLORS

It will sometimes be a considerable strain on you, but you'll be wise to let your youngster play at his own level, progress from one level to another without any pushing from you. The first coloring book your child has will doubtless be a mass of crayon marks, scribbles that pay no attention to the outlines he is supposed to fill in. But he's "drawing" his own way—let him.

At a later stage, he may stick pretty well to filling in the outlines but may make everything the "wrong" color—pink grass, yellow sky, a purple face. Never mind. That's the way he wants it—perhaps the way he sees it—right now. A later stage will bring him to more conventional coloring—and who are we to say that that's "better"? At any rate, don't hurry him and don't correct him—you'll frustrate him, give him the feeling that he can't do anything right.

And, no matter how hard it is, keep your hands off— don't do the job for him. Don't color the picture your way and then say, "See how pretty it is when it's done right?"

Play with him, of course. He loves to have you play with him—if you'll play at his level of development. Let him show *you* the "right" way.

SHARING—AND THE CHILD'S POINT OF VIEW

The concept of sharing with other children comes hard—especially to first children or only children. When your young one first starts playing with other children, you'll find that they are all grabbers, at least if they are aged one and a half to two and a half. A youngster of this age hasn't the slightest idea what you're getting at if you tell him to "share your toys with Johnny" or "let Johnny play with your train for a while." That train is *his,* and the concept of sharing it with someone else is entirely beyond him. If the other child tries to take it away, he'll hang on and howl up a storm. If his mother—don't be guilty of this, will you?—takes it away from him and gives it to the other child, he's bewildered and heartbroken.

Youngsters of around two or so will hang onto their possessions for dear life and fight tooth and nail rather than surrender them. Mothers watching this behavior may be stunned. Believe me, it's normal. And it doesn't mean that your offspring is going to grow up to be a teen-age bully. Of course, if your child looks as if he's about to hit his young friend over the head with the train, you'll have to interfere. But don't make a big fuss. Take him away and get him interested in something else. Later on, when he's a bit older, the concept of sharing—I'll play with your toy and you can play with mine—will dawn on him. Don't tell him what a bad boy he is—he's not. He's just being a normal child acting his age.

Any child over six months old should be given time to himself to learn how to develop his own interests, his own play. It's unnecessary—worse, it's bad for him—for you to be constantly fussing over him, handing him something new to play with the moment he puts down what he was playing with before. You don't want your child to grow up thinking he is the center of the world. This isn't to say you're going to ignore him. But let him initiate things sometimes. Let him play by himself as long as he's willing to. It boils down to this: don't try too hard. It will be good for him and for you.

Attempt to look at things with a child's-eye view as you give your child things to play with or as you play with him. Think about being down on the floor or in a playpen, for example. Do you realize that from his position you see only the undersides of things—the undersides of chair seats, tables, for example. And think of how you look to him—not only enormous, but distorted, elongated.

In the same way, your child sees his play on a scale different from the way you see it from your height. To him, a table is not something to sit at, but something to crawl under —a house, a cave, a retreat. To play on a child's level, you should come down to his level—get down on the floor with him, where you can be, if not his size, more nearly his size. He will appreciate your efforts far more in his own environment than he will in yours, and you can play comfortably together.

Another warning: don't enter into competition with your child. You'll discourage him so that he won't want to try. Yes, you can build a bigger, better tower with his blocks than he can. You can draw a picture better than he can. But don't. You aren't trying to prove that you are older, wiser, more dexterous, more experienced, less awkward than he is. You're *helping* him to learn, not doing his learning for him. Let him teach you—and in doing so, teach himself. Offer suggestions if he seems to want them, help if he seems to want it, but don't do for him what he must do for himself.

COMPARISONS ARE INVIDIOUS

Once again, as I've suggested a number of times throughout this book, don't compare your child with another. Johnny Jones down the street draws a better picture than your child does—more realistic, more properly scaled. So what? Johnny may grow up to be the Rembrandt of his generation, and that isn't going to matter, either. Don't pit your child against another one.

Never say, "Johnny's picture is much better than yours." Say instead, "That's a fine picture—and if you keep on drawing pictures, they'll keep on getting better and better." That's pitting the child against himself, a valuable thing for him to learn: that he can improve himself through practice. Your child knows very early that he cannot be anyone else. He cannot ever be Johnny—but he can be himself, a constantly growing, expanding, improving self.

Later on, when your child is playing unsupervised with other children, the spirit of competition may enter into it—especially with children who have been pushed and goaded by their parents. When that happens and your youngster comes to you and says, "Johnny can run faster than I can," you can smile and say, "Perhaps he can. But he can't run as fast as a car, can he? Or a railroad train? Or a rocket to the moon? And there are many things you do very well, too."

Your child will teach you a lot if you observe him closely. By instinct he does what he needs to do. When he needs exercise, he stretches, kicks, tumbles about on the floor or the grass. When he feels the need to learn skills, he will build, construct, use tools. When he needs information he will ask questions (a seemingly endless stream of questions, as you'll find out, most of them starting with "why"). When he needs love or reassurance he'll climb into your lap and snuggle. When he wants privacy, he will play alone. When he needs experience or discipline, he will "try out" different attitudes and patterns of behavior to see what your reaction to them is.

REGULATED PLAYTIME

As your baby outgrows first his crib, then his playpen, he makes increasing demands on your time. He realizes that you are the source of an almost endless variety of play experiences. You are fun. You make life interesting.

But there are other demands on you. You must now start regulating your time with your little one in such a way that he begins to realize there are things you must do—and also things you want to do—by yourself and that you have a right to some privacy. At the same time he must feel that this attitude on your part in no way diminishes your love for him. And he must know that he *does* have a claim on a portion of your time—certain parts of the day set aside for him.

To help him understand this difference, when his playtimes come don't hesitate, don't make excuses. Play with him, even if there are stacks of dishes waiting to be washed and stacks of clothes waiting to be ironed. Come what may, those times are his, not to be interrupted or cut short. Then he will recognize that you have a right to other times that are yours.

Choose playtimes that are not likely to be interrupted. For a toddler, the best time might be early morning when daddy can participate a bit, too, and again late in the afternoon when mommy's daily chores are done. Later afternoon or early evening are best when a child starts to school—again, with daddy participating if that is possible.

Let the child's needs be your guide. There will be playtimes when he wants to be messy, to slosh around in finger paints or fill the bathtub with water and sail his boats. Sometimes he'll want you to participate, other times to be only an interested spectator, a sort of cheering section while he plays. There will be times when he wants to romp and roughhouse, others when he'll want to sit quietly on your lap while you read him a story.

Very early a child learns to recognize weekends as particularly good times. Then, too, your scheduling will have to be carefully thought out so that you and your husband have time to yourselves. But weekends should also be special times for the child—particularly because daddy is home and can play with him. And when the child gets a little older, weekends will be occasions for special excursions, such as visits to the zoo or to the circus—exciting adventures that your young one will recognize as being undertaken totally for his benefit.

When your child begins to play by himself for any length of time, go to him occasionally, ask how he's doing or suggest a new game or activity if his interest seems to be flagging before he trails out to the kitchen to ask you, "What shall I do *now?*" He'll recognize that you're interested in him even if you aren't playing with him, that you care what he's doing and how he's doing it.

Children of each sex need playtime with the parent of the same sex as well as with the parent of the opposite sex. Boys, playing with their mothers, are laying the foundation for understanding women; girls, playing with their fathers, are laying the foundation for understanding men. When the whole family plays together, the child or children lay the foundation for getting along in a group.

SOME PLAY CAN BE HARMFUL

We've been sounding all along as if playing were just one long round of fun. But there are some kinds of play between parent and child that are harmful and others that can be harmful if carried to extremes. Too much attention is wrong—it makes a child overstimulated, demanding and self-centered. Too little attention is wrong—a child who receives too little attention becomes sad and unresponsive, hardly a human being at all.

It's a favorite pastime of father to toss a baby into the air or to tickle him until he laughs wildly. His excitement on these occasions doesn't grow out of pleasure—it arises from hysteria. Another kind of play that's wrong occurs when the baby is feeling cross (perhaps he's both overtired and teething) and the mother makes a game of letting him vent his anger on her. Play that goes beyond the normal playtime simply because the child demands it is wrong, too. The child loses respect for his parent. Teasing is another poor kind of play. Again, the father may be more likely to do this, although mothers are often guilty, too.

The child is younger, smaller than you and without your fund of experience and knowledge to guide him. With an older child, teasing may take the form of poking fun at him or at something he has made or done. With a little one it may be something as simple as holding out to the baby something he wants and then withdrawing it as he reaches for it.

But most playtimes are joyous times, for both parent and child. Here's an easy test: if you wouldn't like it done to you by someone ten times your size, don't do it to or with the baby. Work by that ground rule and playtime always *will* be joyous.

YOUR CHILD AND HIS PET

A word about one kind of play—with pets. Nearly all children, even very, very young ones, love animals. But they can't be expected to assume all the responsibility of taking care of a pet before they reach the age of six or seven, so the care, training and feeding of any pets will doubtless be your responsibility. Moreover, very small children have no idea of their own strength or the harm it can do or even that little animals can feel pain. Nor do they understand that a hurt animal will retaliate.

Youngsters squeeze toys to hear the toys squeak or cry —they'll squeeze a puppy or a kitten the same way, hoping for the same results. The results are sometimes fatal to the pet, and very often the youngster is bitten or scratched. Unless you are both willing to take care of the pet and to keep it clear of the baby except when you are right on the spot to guard against harm to either one, it's wiser to wait until baby is a little older before getting that puppy or that kitten.

When you get a pet for the child, it is a very good idea not to get a very young animal and to steer clear of fragile toy breeds, such as chihuahuas or toy poodles. You'll find that an older puppy of a medium-sized breed, such as a four- to six-month-old beagle or terrier, or a mixed-breed puppy about that size, will be better able to play with a sometimes-rough youngster and also more inclined, by disposition, to run away if hurt rather than to retaliate. A puppy of that age will be much easier to housebreak, too, than a very young one. Just as young children have very little control of body functions and can't be toilet-trained until they are old enough both to control themselves and to understand why they should, very young puppies are difficult to train.

It's different with kittens. Again, you won't want a fragile, highly bred one—an alley-cat type kitten will be a better choice. However, kittens seem to be born housebroken.

For a very young child a pet to watch is generally better than a pet to have contact with. A pet that is confined, in other words. A bird in a cage, a hamster or gerbil in a cage, a fish in a bowl or a number of fish in a tank—all these are fascinating to a toddler, and the child is safe from the pet, the pet safe from the child.

Here, to finish off the chapter on playing, is a list of playthings and/or play interests that may help you to select toys, activities and experiences for your young one. Bear in mind, though, that each child is an individual—what is broccoli to one child is another's spinach. This list may serve, however, as a rough guide for children in or near each of the age groups listed:

1 month to 8 months
mobiles
soft rubber dolls
rattles
a crib "gym"
bouncer swing
rubber or soft plastic blocks
teething ring
bright blocks with bells in them
soft ball—perhaps one with various textures
squeeze toys

6 months to one year
bells
balls
cork, rubber or soft plastic floating toys for bathtub play
teething rings
nesting blocks
clothes pins
mirror
peg-and-hole blocks
peekaboo
pat-a-cake

1 year to 18 months
pull toys
push toys
small boxes
cuddly animals and dolls
wooden toys big enough to sit on or in
small wooden blocks
chimes
simple jack-in-the-box
toy broom, other "mommy things"
cloth books
ball to roll on the floor

(starts to play hide-and-seek)
nesting blocks of boxes
(starts to sway to, then dance to, music)
a (muffled) drum
a rocking toy to sit in
block shapes to sort and pair

18 months to 2 years
mallet-and-peg toys
balance toy
pots and pans and their lids
wooden animals
wading pool
swing
sandbox and toys to play with in it
music box
picture books
nursery rhymes, simple poetry for children

2 to 2½ years
wooden block train
dolls and doll clothes
doll bed, carriage
pretend ironing board and iron
water-play toys
box with various kinds of catches and latches (daddy can make this easily)
wooden cars, trucks
peg board
nuts and bolts (large enough so they can't be swallowed)
rocking horse
toy telephone
outdoor equipment for climbing and sliding
records to listen to
clay for modeling
large crayons and paper
finger paints
(likes to take things apart and put them together again)
(enjoys a family party or a small party with no more than two other children)

11

Mishaps and Ailments

I'm not a doctor, and so of course I'm not going to make any attempt to offer you medical advice. You must depend on your own personal physician or your clinic for diagnosis and treatment. But I am a mother, and I know the kind of thing that worries mothers—and with reason.

This chapter will deal with some of these, a sort of what to do (and what not to do) until you can get in touch with your doctor—or help, such as your local rescue squad, arrives —especially in emergency situations. Most of these pieces of information apply both to infants and toddlers.

When you're a young mother, especially the young mother of a firstborn, it's very comforting to know in times of emergency that your baby's doctor is only a telephone call away. In fact, mothers caring for their first children, particularly in the early weeks after coming home from the hospital, have a tendency to phone their doctors fairly often, and almost all mothers at all times err on the side of too often rather than not enough.

But you'll find that most doctors are very understanding. They know you are nervous about your abilities and skills in this new job of motherhood. They know how very precious this infant is to you. And they understand that accidents do occur, that babies sometimes develop "symptoms" that are alarming to the mother, even though they may have very little or no meaning medically. Most doctors offer advice something like this: "Call me whenever you feel you should. But take the baby's temperature before you do—that's the first thing I'll ask you." And you will be shown how to take—and read—the baby's temperature with a rectal thermometer.

If at all possible, when you have a baby, have a telephone in your home. If you can't, then be sure you know of a neighbor close by whose telephone will be readily available to you. Or if there is an outdoor phone box near you, be sure of its location and keep a couple of dimes in some special place so that you'll always be able to lay hands on the right change immediately. Be sure that your doctor's telephone number is posted by the phone or in a place where you can find it at once—even if you know it by heart. In times of stress, we're likely to forget the things we "know by heart."

It's a good idea to have other important numbers posted, too—those of the emergency medical center, if your town has one; the poison control center, if your town has one; the police and fire department emergency numbers and the number of the hospital nearest you. If you are really in trouble and all else fails, dial O on your telephone for the operator, give her your name and address and tell her the nature of the emergency—she'll get help to you.

The first thing to do if a problem or an emergency occurs is for you to *keep calm*. The little one can't do anything to help himself—you are in charge, and you have to do the helping or the getting of help. Take a deep breath and survey the situation to determine what has happened and what must be done. Call the doctor. Then take whatever action you can—and is necessary—until the doctor can be located or until he comes or tells you to bring the child to him.

You will want to call the doctor, and to follow his advice, in these situations:

* When the child's temperature (and especially an infant's) registers over 100.4 degrees on a rectal thermometer.
* When the child is pale and his lips, skin and nails are blue, although it is not cold enough to warrant such symptoms.
* When the white areas of the eyes take on a yellow color.
* When the child seems drowsy for no reason (not just because he's sleepy) and/or if he seems to be having difficulty in breathing or swallowing.
* When the child is vomiting—not just an infant's normal spitting up—or has diarrhea with many loose stools, or if bowel movement is black, white or contains blood.
* When the child has a rash you cannot identify (such as diaper rash), especially if there is accompanying fever.
* When the child urinates more frequently than usual, especially if urination is accompanied by discomfort or by bleeding.
* When there are rapid back-and-forth movements of the eyes.
* When a child's ear has been injured or is draining or looks puffy, or when the child says his ear pains or, if he is too young to tell you, when he cries out as if in pain or hits at his ear with his hand, or when there appears to be a disturbance in hearing.
* When the child is listless for more than a few hours, especially if he refuses liquids.
* When the child has an open wound or an open sore.
* When the child's nose bleeds.
* When the child is excessively irritable even though there seems to be no cause for it (he's not tired, or should not be tired, for example).

* When the child has a cough that produces blood or is accompanied by fever or sounds croupy (he makes a choking noise).
* When the child breathes rapidly and/or with a raspy sound, particularly if he looks distressed even though he is properly rested.
* When there are white spots on the insides of his cheeks that cannot be wiped off.
* When he exhibits any sort of unusual, peculiar behavior—such as frequent blank stares, for example.
* When there is an accident or other emergency, such as the swallowing (or poking into the ear or nose) of a foreign object, particularly a sharp object or a poisonous substance.
* When there is bleeding from any body opening.

There are occasions on which a mother wants to—or, indeed, will need to—take some action above and beyond phoning the doctor in the interval between calling for help and the arrival of help. I know that "Keep your head!" is easy to say and very hard to do in an emergency situation. When the emergency is over and the child has received proper care, you can have hysterics if you want to—but not until then!

There may come a time when everything that gets done will be up to you to do. Accidents do happen, and sometimes they occur in places where a doctor or a hospital emergency room is not immediately available. Here are some guidelines. Use them as a basis for asking your doctor questions—in advance—so that you will know what to do in case of an emergency. We'll start with some of the simpler accident-emergencies and then cover the more serious ones.

* *Scrapes:* Use wet cotton or gauze to wipe off gently, using clean water and soap. Apply a non-stick sterile dressing. (Whenever the skin is broken, and in the case of burns even when skin does not appear to be broken, the doctor may want to protect the child against tetanus—follow his advice.)
* *Bruises:* Apply cold compresses (don't put ice di-

rectly on the skin) for about half an hour. If the skin is broken, treat it as you would a cut.

* *Cuts:* Wash small cuts with soap and clean water. Cover with a sterile dressing. In the case of a large cut, apply dressing and press down firmly to stop the bleeding. If you are in some place where no sterile dressing is available, use a piece of the cleanest clothing on you or the child to apply pressure to stop bleeding. Don't use a tourniquet unless you cannot stop the bleeding in any other way—if you must use one, loosen at intervals. Do not use any antiseptic on a cut, large or small, until the doctor has seen it and directs you to do so.

* *Puncture wounds:* Call the doctor, describe the wound and do as he directs you.

* *Slivers:* Wash with clean water and soap. Remove the sliver, if easily accessible, with a pair of tweezers. If the sliver is large or deeply embedded, follow your doctor's directions.

* *Burns, minor:* If burned area is on arm or hand, leg or foot, immerse the extremity in cold water. Cold, wet packs or an ice bag may be applied if the burn is in a position where it can't be immersed in cold water. Cover with a nonadhesive dressing. In an emergency, kitchen plastic film—Saran Wrap or the like—can be used as a nonadhesive covering.

* *Burns, extensive:* Keep the child in a flat position. Remove clothing over burned area unless it is stuck to the burn—if stuck, leave it in place. Cover with clean cloth. Keep patient warm. If doctor cannot come at once, get the patient to hospital emergency center. Do not use greases, ointments or powders on a burn. Electric burns with accompanying shock may require artificial respiration (see below).

* *Burns, chemical:* Wash thoroughly with water. Follow doctor's directions.

* *Fractures:* Adult bones generally break, but young children's bones are more likely to bend and splin-

ter—what is known as a "green-stick fracture." Suspect fracture when the injured part looks deformed. Do not move the child if a fracture of the leg or back is suspected. Wait for the arrival of doctor or rescue squad.

* *Sprains:* Elevate the injured part and apply cold compresses for half an hour. If there is considerable swelling, do not allow the child to use the injured part until the doctor has examined it.

* *Eyes, foreign bodies:* If you can see and easily reach the object, remove it with a moistened piece of cotton rolled between the fingers until of proper size. If not, wait until the doctor comes to you or take the child to the doctor. If there is pain in the eye, bandage it shut until the doctor can examine it.

* *Eyes, chemicals:* Flush out with large amounts of plain water immediately.

* *Nosebleeds:* With the child in sitting position, have him blow out from the nose any blood or blood clot. Insert into the bleeding nostril a small wad of cotton moistened with water or peroxide and press firmly with your finger on the outside of the nose for five minutes. If bleeding has not stopped, continue pressure and follow doctor's directions.

* *Fainting:* If a child loses consciousness, keep him in a flat position while waiting for the doctor or rescue squad. Loosen clothing. Keep patient warm and his mouth clear. Don't give him anything to swallow.

* *Injuries to the head:* Keep the patient absolutely quiet until the doctor is able to advise you.

* *Choking:* If child cannot breathe, turn him face down over your knee and hit his back firmly between the shoulder blades in an effort to jar the object out of his windpipe. If he can breathe and is merely uncomfortable, wait for the doctor or emergency squad.

* *Artificial respiration:* You may never need to use mouth-to-mouth or mouth-to-nose artificial respiration—but you should know the technique in case

of drowning or electric shock. The time to learn the technique is before an emergency happens—to understand it so well that you can apply it easily and, if necessary, for a long period of time. Ask your doctor to show you how to use mouth-to-mouth or mouth-to-nose artificial respiration or learn the technique from your local Red Cross or from classes conducted by your local rescue squad. The important things to remember: begin at once and do not stop until the patient is breathing.

* *Poison, swallowed:* Call the doctor, a hospital, poison control center or rescue unit immediately. Tell the person who answers what the substance was that the child swallowed. Follow the instructions that will be given you until help arrives. You may be told to dilute the poison by giving water or to make the patient vomit—or, in the case of corrosive poisons or petroleum derivatives, or if the patient is having convulsions, *not* to make the patient vomit. In any case, follow the instructions you are given to the letter.

* *Poison, fumes or gases:* Have someone else call the doctor, rescue squad, hospital or poison control center while you get the child to clean, fresh air, loosen his clothing and, if he is not breathing, start artificial respiration at once and do not stop until patient is breathing well or help arrives.

* *Poison, in the eye:* Gently wash out eye immediately with clean water—or use milk if no water is available; do this for five minutes with eyelid held open while someone else calls for help.

* *Poison, on the skin:* Wash immediately in large amounts of water, using soap if it is available. Remove clothing with any of the substance on it. Call for help or have someone else do so.

* *Bites, snake:* Keep the child as quiet as possible —do not let him walk. Transport him as rapidly as possible to doctor or hospital. En route, or while awaiting transportation, apply suction to the wound

with suction cup or mouth. Give artificial respiration if child stops breathing.

* *Bites, insect:* Bites from scorpions and some spiders are dangerous; in addition some people have allergic reactions, sometimes very serious, to the stings of such insects as bees, wasps and hornets. Do not let the child walk or exercise. Use any cold substance available to place on the area to relieve pain. Get prompt help for the child. If he stops breathing, use artificial respiration.

* *Bites, animal:* There is always the possibility that a wild animal—such as a skunk, a bat, etc.—may have rabies, and the possibility that a dog may also have the disease, even though he is someone's pet. If at all possible, the animal should be captured—this is a business for experts, not amateurs—and brought in for observation. Call for help and wash the wound gently but thoroughly with soap and water.

SICKNESS AND ACCIDENT

If you have policed your yard and babyproofed your house, as we discussed in Chapter Seven, you have removed many of the causes for accident. However, you should not think that your little one will never have an accident or never be sick. Young ones do catch colds, have respiratory infections, climb on things and promptly fall off them—there are always certain troubles in childhood.

Regular habits, good nutrition, lots of loving care and reasonable avoidance of exposure to infection whenever possible are important in maintaining your child's good health. Some of the diseases that in grandparents', parents', even in your own, time of childhood took a heavy toll have been conquered by immunization. Your doctor will tell you on what schedule he wants to give your baby these all-important shots. If you cannot afford to have them given by a private physician, a health-department clinic will give them at little or no cost.

Here's a guide, to help you know, in general, what to expect. Most well babies, by the time they are five months old, have received three injections of combined diphtheria, tetanus and pertussis (whooping cough) vaccine—that is called D.T.P.—and have had two or three doses of oral polio vaccine. At one year or thereabouts, a shot of measles vaccine is given. Smallpox vaccination usually comes sometime during baby's second year unless there is some reason for giving it earlier or postponing it—your doctor or clinic will decide.

There are also vaccines for mumps, German measles and typhoid—the doctor will decide if and when to give those. When the baby is about one year old, he will be given a skin test for tuberculosis. Booster shots will be given at various stages. When some of these shots are given, your child may develop a slight fever or otherwise feel mildly unwell. The doctor or nurse will tell you what to expect so that you'll be prepared for the reaction.

DON'T BE AFRAID TO ASK QUESTIONS

When your child is sick and you take him to the doctor or the doctor comes to the house, ask questions about anything that bothers you. How long will he be sick? What's wrong with him? Is it serious? What do the terms mean that the doctor has used if you don't understand them? Have confidence in your doctor and rely on what he tells you. If you don't have confidence in him, perhaps he is not the right doctor for you.

A child who is only slightly ill—who has a cold, for example—will generally pattern his behavior after yours. If you behave as if he's very sick, so will he. It's up to you to keep calm, to treat the matter seriously but not gravely, so that the child will not be frightened. Be calm and friendly, make his meals appetizing (he probably won't have much of an appetite, so don't worry if he eats very little) and follow the doctor's instructions.

12

Travel Is Broadening

The way we Americans travel, there's every chance that you'll be taking some kind of trip while your child is small. Perhaps it will be a vacation or a trip to visit relatives (must show off the little one to grandma and grandpa if they can't come to see him!) or possibly a move caused by your husband's transfer to a new job some distance away. Maybe you'll be going only a short distance or perhaps across the country or even overseas.

Whatever the length of the journey, you'll find that some careful advance planning can make the trip a truly enjoyable experience—not only for you and your child but also for the other people who are in the plane, train, bus or car, not to mention the people whom you go to visit. By thinking and preparing ahead, you can make travel very simple and easy—and the simpler you make it, the easier and more pleasant you'll find it to be!

BABY'S PHYSICAL NEEDS

If your youngster is still just a young baby, planning will center around attending to his physical needs, and not much

FROM Gerber®

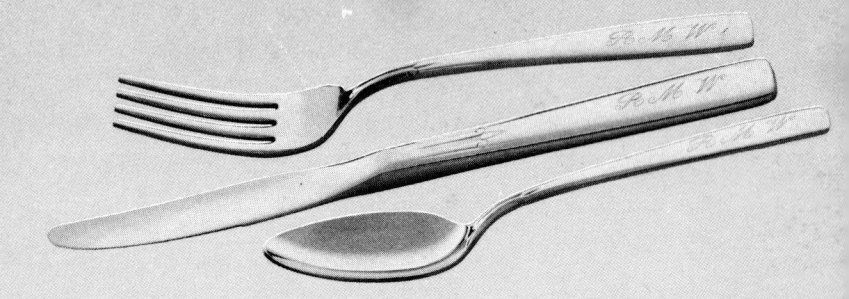

PRACTICAL
"Child's own Tableware"
IN STUNNING STAINLESS

- Child's initials on all three pieces to be his very own for life
- Proportioned to fit any child's hands for stimulating self-feeding
- A thoughtful, personalized gift that never wears out but becomes a lasting keepsake.
- Beautifully polished stainless steel for easy-care and life-time durability
- Lovely Oneida pattern in clean, classic design

Price per engraved set
$2.49

**Gerber Products Company
Department B.U.B.
Fremont, Michigan 49412**

Dear Sirs:

I want to order ___ Toddler Tableware set(s). For each set ordered, I am enclosing $2.49 (check or money order, made payable to Gerber Products Co.). I understand Gerber will handle all postage and mailing anywhere in the continental United States.

CHILD'S INITIALS ☐ ☐ ☐

PLEASE MAIL MY ORDER TO:

NAME _____
(Please Print Plainly)

ADDRESS _____

CITY _____ STATE _____ ZIP CODE _____

Allow 4 weeks for delivery. Offer expires July 31, 1974.
(If expired, please write Gerber for new offers.)

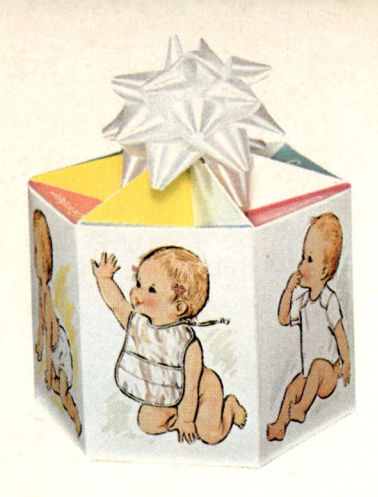

Looking for a "New Baby" gift?

Gerber Babywear Basics

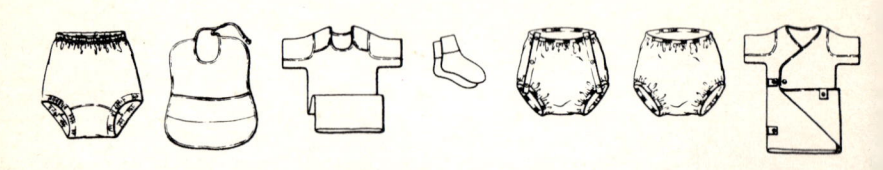

Gerber has the answer with a gift assortment of famous-for-quality Gerber babywear. Shipped complete in an attractive, colorful gift package topped off with a bow, the babywear assortment is perfect for that shower or new-baby gift—perfect for your own use, too!

The gift package contains seven different Gerber garments and is available in three different size assortments. Included are snap-on and pull-on vinyl pants, snap-on and pull-on cotton shirts, cotton training pants, nylon stretch socks and a vinyl bib.

As a special offer to readers, we are making it available for $3.50

**Gerber Products Company
Department B.U.B.
Fremont, Michigan 49412**

Dear Sirs:

I want to order ____ seven-piece babywear kit(s). For each kit ordered, I am enclosing $3.50 (check or money order, made payable to Gerber Products Co.). I understand Gerber will handle all postage and mailing anywhere in the continental United States.

Check (✓) size desired: ☐ Birth to 18 lbs.   ☐ 19–24 lbs.   ☐ 25–34 lbs.

PLEASE MAIL MY ORDER TO:

NAME _____
(Please Print Plainly)

ADDRESS _____

CITY _____ STATE _____ ZIP CODE _____

Allow 4 weeks for delivery. Offer expires July 31, 1974.
(If expired, please write Gerber for new offers.)

concern need be given to keeping him amused. You'll find that it's a very good idea to have disposable diapers if you aren't already using these handy items. The disposable diapers speak for themselves—they free you of the problem of coping with wet or dirty diapers on the trip. Plastic nursers eliminate the risk of broken bottles—which can be dangerous, messy and very frustrating when you have a hungry baby on your hands and the broken bottle contained the last prepared formula you were carrying with you. (Somehow, with the cussedness of inanimate objects with which we're all so familiar, it's always the last available bottle that gets broken or spilled!)

There are several ways of preparing and carrying formula with you when you are traveling—choose the most convenient for you, depending on the facilities you will have for preparing formula en route and how long you will be away from adequate refrigeration. Check the railroad or airline in advance to see if they can refrigerate formula for you and how many bottles they are able to accept.

The simplest thing to do is to carry ready-to-feed formula with you if your doctor says this is all right in your baby's case. If you're going to feed him ready-mixed formula on the trip, you should start him on it well in advance, however, because new foods, no matter how great they are, are sometimes upsetting to a baby's digestive system. These formulas really are wonderful—they come in disposable containers and they don't have to be refrigerated. The whole works can be thrown away after a feeding—there's nothing to wash or sterilize.

If you can't get or can't use ready-prepared formula, and you are going to be on your journey for less than twenty-four hours, prepare your regular formula at home before you leave and carry it with you in a picnic refrigerator in your car or use the refrigeration service provided by train or plane. Carry it in separate bottles or in one large bottle. In the latter case, you'll have to carry nursing bottles, nipples and a funnel, as well as soap and brush to wash the bottles and nipples after they are used, if you don't take along enough bottles to last through the trip.

In the car, using a carry-along icebox, you'll be better off carrying the formula in enough separate bottles to last you. Be sure the bottles of formula are well chilled before you start. Pack the bottles in ice and wrap the whole refrigerator in at least ten layers of newspaper, which is a great insulating material. If the trip is a short one, carry a couple of chilled bottles in an insulated bottle carrier—again, make doubly sure by wrapping well in newspaper.

The simplest—and therefore the best—solution, however, if at all possible, is to use ready-prepared formula, no matter what mode of travel you are using.

IN THE FAMILY CAR ... AND OTHER CARRIERS

When you're traveling in the family car, you may want to make a stop once each day at a shopping center to buy disposable diapers and prepared formula. Such a stop gives you and the driver a break, allows you to stretch your legs and makes it unnecessary to carry large amounts of supplies with you. While you're at it, buy fresh sweet rolls for tomorrow's breakfast, if you like—it does seem that the more you stay out of restaurants with a possibly fretful youngster, the pleasanter your trip will be. So when you pack for baby's meals, do a little packing for the adults, too. Carry along instant coffee, sugar, powdered cream substitutes and disposable cups and spoons. A noonday picnic is sometimes a good idea, too—make your daily stop early and pick up milk, sandwiches, fruit and perhaps packaged cookies for a middle-of-the-day meal.

For the baby on solids, small jars of baby food and a supply of plastic spoons make good sense. You can warm the food in an auto bottle warmer if you don't like to serve it at "room temperature"—although many authorities say nowadays that warming isn't necessary. Or you can ask a restaurant waitress or the dining car steward or the plane stewardess to warm the food for you. All these people are used to such requests and are generally very accommodating.

In a train you can warm food or a bottle yourself by putting the container into warm water run into a washroom basin. In planning for a trip, don't feel it necessary to carry along everything that the baby usually gets. (Skip potatoes for the duration, for instance, or scrambled eggs or anything else that will be hard to come by.) Feed the baby entirely from jars and don't attempt to keep any leftovers from one feeding to the next. Open fresh jars for each meal.

It's not wise to give your baby or young child water from a faucet while you're traveling, even if he is well past the age where water is usually boiled for him. Chances are that drinking tap water may cause bowel upsets. You'll find it a very good idea to use bottled sterilized distilled water. You might get the little one used to it (it's absolutely tasteless and probably will seem very flat to you) for a few days before starting out on the trip. Water is another one of the things you can buy along the way as you need it—there's no necessity for loading down the car with jugs of water.

The younger the baby, the easier the trip, since the motion of the car will serve to lull him. The best place for a baby to travel is in the back seat, in a sturdy car bed. A word of warning: it *has* been proven that the front seat, with baby riding in your arms or in your lap, is the most dangerous part of the car for a baby in the event of accident. Of course, you probably won't have an accident—but why take chances with something as precious as your little one? Snuggle him down in back.

Incidentally, when you have a youngster in the back seat, it's wise to keep the rear deck free of any objects that are heavy or that have sharp or hard edges. A sudden stop can send them crashing down onto the baby, with the possibility of serious injury.

You might consider turning your car's entire back seat into a padded play area for your youngster. There are a number of items on the market for this purpose—seat fences, car-seat playpens and specially constructed mattresses, to name a few. And of course you can easily improvise your own. You can put two suitcases in the rear foot area to form a base, then pad them to seat height and cover them with a playpen pad. This will create a firm yet soft base, and with small pillows and a blanket you'll have a safe, comfortable nest for your active six-to-nine-month-old who is unhappy in the confines of a car bed or a car seat. If you have a four-door car, remember to lock those back doors!

TRAVEL LIGHT

While you'll find that there are many things which you absolutely must take along, you'll discover also that the lighter you can travel, the easier and more enjoyable time you'll have. You will want to take baby's toys, of course, but you needn't take everything he might conceivably want. Limit your choice to just a few small, easily packed, tried-and-true favorites. Remember, the trip itself is going to be a distraction, making his toys less necessary. And don't give him everything you've brought along at once. Hold back one or two favorites for a time when he is tired and bored.

By the same token, rather than crowding valuable space by taking along the crib, playpen, stroller and so on, it's a good idea to budget so you can rent them at your destination. If you are visiting friends or relatives, they may have all such needed items or will be able to borrow them. It's a good idea to check this point in advance.

One smart young mother I know tells me that she packs each outfit for her youngster in a separate plastic bag—socks, underwear, overalls and shirt (or dress) and sweater. That way she doesn't need to hunt all through the suitcase to assemble the outfit. She says she now does the same with her own outfits and that it makes packing both easy and neat. She also advises choosing drip-dry clothing for children with simple zip or snap closings and leaving at home the outfits which are difficult to launder or to put on, regardless of how cute they may be.

If your trip is going to require one or more overnight stops (and it's a poor idea to drive straight through), plan to stop at a reasonable hour. (Make a pact with your husband in advance that it will be the hour of the day, not the number of miles traveled in a day, that determines each afternoon's stopping time.)

And it's *very* wise, especially during peak vacation times, to make reservations ahead so that you're sure of having a room. Few things are more worrisome and frustrating than being told by place after place that it is filled and having to drive and drive when you're already so tired you feel you can't last another mile. You'll finally settle for unattractive quarters—or, at the other extreme, a luxury unit larger and far more expensive than you need and can really afford. Many of the big chains of motels will make free reservations ahead for you with other members of their chain. They also provide free cribs, as a rule, make no charge for children under the age of twelve years, can supply baby-sitters—why, they often even will welcome the family dog as well!

OTHER TIPS FOR TODDLERS

Another girl-on-the-go says to tell you, whatever you do, to let your toddler explore the room thoroughly upon arrival. It may be tempting to let a sleeping youngster sleep and quietly go on to bed yourselves. Just as sure as you do, he'll wake up in the middle of the night and start exploring then and there!

Traveling with a toddler *is* more of a problem than with a baby, but he's more interested in everything that is going on around him, so you'll find that it is more rewarding, too. That same girl-on-the-go also advises taking along something for a between-meals snack, such as crackers or simple cookies.

Perhaps you have the problem of a child who is famished *until* you get to a restaurant and his meal is put before him, at which time he loses his appetite—until you are back in the car, miles from anywhere, that is! When you order, decide on food that you can carry along for him to eat later. Carry small plastic bags with you or ask the waitress for a bag or foil. This happens so often that restaurants catering to travelers are used to it, so there's no need for you to feel self-conscious about doing it.

A plastic tablecloth is a big help when you are traveling with a youngster. You can use it many different ways. It can protect mattresses against bed-wetting and safeguard anything on which you change the baby's diaper. It can cover the carpet when you are feeding the baby or when he is playing on the floor.

It is important to take along the toilet seat or the potty chair your child is accustomed to using at home to avoid toilet problems.

Travel by bus, plane or train creates more problems,

for you can take along much less. On the other hand, the trip usually takes much less time, too, and porters and stewardesses are helpful. Now, how to simplify this kind of travel?

First of all, here is where you *really* must travel light. A baby, medium-sized bag and over-shoulder bag are all you can safely manage by yourself if you are traveling alone (and it's best to assume that you will have to manage by yourself). Of course, you can check additional luggage through to your destination.

Start in plenty of time. You'll find that your trip will be much more enjoyable if you get to the airport or terminal early and are relaxed and able to get aboard in time to get a window seat close to an exit than if you just barely make connections, are tense and worried over your crying baby and then find that all the best seats are already taken.

In air travel, have a bottle or a pacifier for your baby to suck during the takeoff and landing—sucking and swallowing help ease ear discomfort if it occurs, due to pressure.

Incidentally, you should never travel with a sick youngster if you can possibly avoid it or with a child who has been exposed to any communicable disease until after the incubation period has passed. This is especially true if you are going by air. Even a case of sniffles, a cough or nasal congestion might turn into a serious problem in the pressurized cabin of a plane in those rare instances of sudden ascent or descent. Postpone your trip or go by a different means of transportation if there is any sign of a cold. Even adult airline personnel must obey this rule.

With just a little advance planning and a relaxed attitude, you'll find that travel with a baby can be a real pleasure, and of course, you'll make new friends as people admire your charming, well-behaved youngster!

13

Some Ideas

Up until now we've been discussing the average baby—healthy, with no real problems—but of course babies are like people of all ages; some do have problems. Since I am in the baby food industry, naturally it is dietary problems that are most familiar to me.

Babies are—quite rarely, fortunately—intolerant of many of even the most basic foods: wheat, corn, citrus fruits, eggs and even that seemingly indispensable food, milk. These intolerances occur often enough that our Gerber nutritionists have made special lists of the Gerber baby foods and formulas that are safe for the little ones with dietary problems. These lists, plus a comprehensive list, *Ingredients in Gerber Baby Foods,* are frequently revised and are free for the asking. However, they do apply only to Gerber products—other brands may contain somewhat different ingredients. When feeding problems of any sort exist, help is available to you from baby food companies. Ask your questions and you'll receive answers.

Bear in mind, if your baby does develop an intolerance, that no one food is absolutely essential. Calcium can be gained from sources other than milk, protein from foods besides eggs. True, it narrows choice, but there are still many excellent foods available. Your youngster can be quite healthy and make excellent progress without certain food categories—as he most certainly will not if he continues to consume whatever gives him trouble.

But perhaps your baby doesn't actually have an intolerance. Perhaps he is just a finicky eater, possibly because of illness robbing him of a hearty appetite, possibly because he is just one of those individuals who isn't terribly interested in eating. So you will find it necessary to tempt him. How do you go about this without fussing over mealtimes?

Well, there again our excellent home economists have come up with some great ideas—not to mention additional inspirations offered by mothers who either had to tempt faint appetites or who simply enjoyed adding a gourmet touch to baby diets.

Beet Borsch: Combine 1 container Gerber Strained Beets with 1 teaspoon sugar and ¼ teaspoon salt. Beat 1 egg yolk. Combine with ½ cup whole milk and the beet mixture. Heat and simmer 5 minutes. Add 1 tablespoon lemon juice. Serve hot or cold. Makes 2 servings.

Cream of Vegetable Soup: Melt 1 tablespoon fat. Add ¼ cup any Gerber cereal and blend well. Add 1 cup whole milk and cook until thickened and smooth. Add 1 container of any Gerber strained vegetable or ½ cup of any Gerber junior vegetable. Add salt to taste, and heat. Makes 2 large or 3 small servings. Note: For increased nutritive value add 2 tablespoons of any Gerber strained or junior meat.

Carrot-and-Cheese Soufflé: Melt 2 tablespoons butter or margarine. Blend in 4 teaspoons any Gerber cereal and a few grains of salt. Add ¼ cup whole milk and cook over low heat, stirring constantly, until thick and smooth. Add 1/3 cup grated mild cheese and 1 container Gerber Strained Carrots. Separate 2 eggs. Beat yolks lightly and stir gradually into carrot mixture. Beat egg whites until stiff and fold in. Spoon into greased baking cups or small casserole. Place in a pan of hot water and bake in a preheated 325° oven about 50 minutes or until center is firm. Makes 3 large or 5 small servings.

Mock Chicken Legs: Melt 1 tablespoon butter or margarine. Add 1 tablespoon all-purpose flour and blend well. Add ¼ cup whole milk and ½ chicken bouillon cube. Cook over low heat, stirring constantly, until thick. Remove from heat. Add 1 container Gerber Junior Beef and 1 container Gerber Junior Veal or Pork. Cool. Shape into "drumsticks" around skewers. Roll in dried bread crumbs. Brush with melted butter or margarine. Bake in preheated 375° oven until brown. Makes 6 small or 3 large drumsticks.

Veal Mousse: Soften 2 tablespoons unflavored gelatin in 2 tablespoons cold water. Beat 2 egg yolks slightly and combine with ½ cup whole milk. Add ½ chicken bouillon cube. Cook in top of double boiler until thickened. Remove from heat. Add softened gelatin, stirring until dissolved. Add 2 containers Gerber Junior Veal. Whip until stiff ¼ cup chilled undiluted evaporated milk. Fold into veal mixture. Pour into lightly oiled small loaf pan and chill until firm. Makes 4 to 5 servings.

Spicy Applesauce Molds: Soften 1 envelope plain gelatin in ¼ cup cold water. Heat 2 containers Gerber Strained Applesauce. Add 2 tablespoons red cinnamon candies and stir until dissolved. Add gelatin and stir until dissolved. Stir in 2 tablespoons lemon juice and 2 tablespoons sugar. Pour into lightly oiled molds and chill until firm. Makes 3 to 4 servings.

Fruit-Salad Dressing: Combine 2 tablespoons salad oil, 1 container Gerber Strained Plums with Tapioca, ¼ cup lemon juice, 1 tablespoon sugar, ¾ teaspoon salt. Chill. Shake well before serving. Makes ¾ cup.

Apricot Surprise Pudding: Cream 2 tablespoons shortening. Gradually add 1/3 cup sugar, creaming well. Add 2 egg yolks and beat until mixture is fluffy. Add 2 tablespoons sifted all-purpose flour and blend well. Add 1 container Gerber Strained Apricots with Tapioca, 1 tablespoon lemon juice and ½ teaspoon grated lemon rind. Mix well. Add ¾ cup milk slowly, and stir until well blended. Beat 2 egg whites stiff but not dry. Fold apricot mixture into egg whites. Pour mixture in greased custard cups. Place in a pan of hot water and bake in a preheated 250° oven 35 minutes. Makes 6 servings.

We have many more such recipes that we will be glad to send you. Just write to Gerber Products Company, Dept. BUB, Fremont, Michigan 49412.

BABIES ARE OUR BUSINESS

And although, as our company motto goes, *Babies Are Our Business,* sometimes grown-ups find strained baby foods useful, too. The smooth texture and the low fiber and fat content, not to mention the mild seasonings that are needed by babies, are frequently found to be necessary in some adult special diets. Many digestive disturbances call for finely divided, bland foods. Also, the fine texture is very helpful when problems arise in chewing or swallowing, caused by dental extractions, jaw fractures or throat obstructions. Sometimes these special diets may need to be continued for quite a long time, and without careful thought and planning such diets become so monotonous that patients find it very difficult to stick to the diet.

Baby foods have been found to be an economical and convenient solution to such problems. They are also excellent for older people who live alone, even if they have no dietary problems. The small containers are ideal for this use, as they allow a wide variety without waste. And it is quite simple to adapt baby foods to adult use. They can be prepared quite quickly, even with limited cooking facilities.

Our talented Gerber Products nutritionists have developed many recipes that the whole family can enjoy. If you would like to have some of these recipes, just write and ask for Family Recipes Featuring Gerber Products.

There's more to making mealtime pleasant than just the food itself. If you have a child whose appetite must be tempted, you'll find it wise to arrange an attractive tray or table. A flower or a trinket or special holiday decorations are helpful. Small portions (with the promise of second helpings, if desired) encourage poor appetites. Tidying up the child and his surroundings just before mealtime often seems to do wonders to increase anticipation and pleasure in eating.

Birthday time—but your youngster isn't allowed to have cake? Put tiny candle in his baby food dessert. He'll love them.

If any family member who's on a special diet is eating at the table with the rest of the family, it's a very good idea to make his food look as much like that which everyone else is eating as possible. Serving plates before they are brought to the table is often helpful. And the old rule of keeping table conversation pleasant is doubly important when someone is dieting. And speaking of conversation, it's wise not to talk about the special diet or conditions that make it necessary any more than you can help.

And now—eat and enjoy, and may you and yours never *need* a special diet!

14

Questions Many Mothers Ask

Question: I don't want to be nosy, but are you a real person or is "Mrs. Gerber" just a sort of trade name? That is, I know that a good many companies do have a representative using a fictitious company name.
Answer: I'm happy to report that I'm very much alive and real. I'm the mother of five, who have presented me with eighteen wonderful grandchildren. That was the count at the time this was written!
Question: How did it all begin, the Gerber baby food business? Did you start out to make baby food or just get into it?
Answer: My husband and father-in-law operated a cannery, and when Dan saw what I went through straining vegetables (especially peas!) for our babies, he thought there must be some better way: to start with fresher produce and get more food value—and incidentally make life a lot easier for mothers. So he put his expert know-how to work on the problem. He succeeded so well that more and more mothers wanted some, so after a great deal of experimenting and reading studies by pediatricians and baby clinics, the Gerber company put its baby foods on the market. After that, the

company just grew and grew, one thing leading to another.
Question: I've heard about the tests you do on your new products. Could my baby and I take part in a test?
Answer: It's possible that you could. We don't like to use the same panels of babies time after time, so we sometimes need new "testers." (Besides, babies *do* have a way of growing up!) Just send in your baby's name, sex and birthdate (and your own name and address, of course), and if possible we'll be in touch with you with a test suited to your baby's age. Incidentally, it isn't just our new products we test—we're constantly working to make our old favorites even better.
Question: My baby seems so hairy! I worried about it until I found, in talking to other mothers, that their babies have or had hair all down the sides of their faces and on their shoulders and backs. We've been wondering about it but never seem to get around to asking the doctors—or if we do, they just kid us and tell us it isn't permanent. Do *you* know anything about it?
Answer: Yes, all that extra hair is called "lanugo," and as the doctors told you and your friends, it isn't permanent. Generally it is gone by the time the baby is two months old. The idea seems to be that it protects a newborn's tender skin. It isn't so noticeable if blond, but I agree, it can be startling when the hair is dark.
Question: My mother frets because my baby isn't wearing a bellyband. She has me wondering, too—if babies always used to wear bellybands in the past, why don't they wear them nowadays? Or is it just my doctor who is being modern?
Answer: Trust your doctor! Doctors now are in general agreement that a baby's navel will heal better if it is left uncovered. The bellyband sometimes got wet with urine or perspiration, then would tighten up and keep out the air which helps to dry the navel.
Question: My baby's head is shaped so funny—just like an egg! Will it always be like that? Is there anything I can do?
Answer: Yes, relax and don't worry about it. Babies' heads are quite flexible, to make the birth process easier for both mother and baby. Often the head is "molded" as it makes its way through the birth canal. However, the head will soon assume its normal shape, without anything being done about it.

Question: At first my baby's skin was so pretty and pink. Now it has a funny yellowish tinge. My doctor told me not to worry about it, but I can't help wondering what causes it.
Answer: This is what's called "normal new-baby jaundice," and about 50 percent of all babies do get it on the second or third day. It's caused by the breaking down of some excess blood cells which the baby needed during your pregnancy but no longer requires. It will disappear soon, and your baby will be pink and pretty again.

Question: My baby has red marks on her face and neck. Can anything be done about them? Are they caused by anything I did or didn't do?
Answer: Many babies do have what are sometimes referred to as "port-wine stains"—their skin is so thin and tender that during birth the blood capillaries break down and show through. Sometimes they completely disappear in a matter of weeks, months at the most. Ask your doctor about treatment if the marks do not disappear.

Question: My sister and I have babies about the same age, and we've been curious as to why my son's navel bulges out and her little girl's dents in. Can you satisfy our curiosity?
Answer: Many babies—especially boys—do have navels that "pop out" or "pout." The bulge is caused because muscles in the wall of the stomach are still weak. Another reason may be that new babies do not have much of a fatty layer. As they fill out, and muscles become stronger, the navel will look perfectly normal. Sometimes it takes only a short time, but often it will take two years or more. However, it is very seldom a cause for worry.

Question: I know my baby is normal, but I keep wondering, why are newborn babies' legs so bowed? Feet bluish? And why is his chin so small?
Answer: Babies just take time to "get in shape"—parts of them are less finished than others at birth. The chin and puny-looking legs you mentioned are good examples. Hands and feet often have a bluish tinge because a baby's circulatory system hasn't really gotten going at its best.

Question: My baby has a rash on his neck. What causes it? I keep him very clean.
Answer: Most new babies do get rashes at one time or another,

for their skin is extremely sensitive. Rashes come and go and usually are due to some slight irritation. Cleanliness helps—but you might take into account that he might be sensitive to something in the soap you use; you could try other soaps, lotions, etc., if rashes persist. (And, of course, if the rash does persist, you'll be talking about it to your doctor—I am just offering ideas, born of long experience, for what they're worth.) Continue to bathe carefully, powder lightly, and you might occasionally give the irritated area an "air bath."

Question: My baby has never had diaper rash, and I want to be sure he doesn't get it. Can you give me some tips for avoiding it?

Answer: It's simple—and you are probably already doing the right things. Change him often. Never leave a soiled diaper on any longer than necessary. Every so often you might let him go without any diaper at all for about 15 minutes. Be sure diapers are completely free of soaps or detergents (this is routine with diaper services).

Question: Speaking of diapers, how many and what kind are best for my baby?

Answer: New babies use between 90 and 100 a week. Of course, if you are laundering your own rather than using a diaper service, you won't need that many. Buy the softest ones you can find—gauze, bird's-eye or prefold, whichever you choose.

Question: How much clothing should I put on my baby during hot weather?

Answer: Just as little as possible. You'll find that a short-sleeved shirt and a diaper—or just a diaper—will be plenty on the hottest days. Keep your youngster comfortable and don't overdress him. Cotton is a good hot-weather material, for it absorbs moisture easily and quickly.

Question: There is so much about breast-feeding nowadays, but I don't know. Should I try to nurse my baby if I really don't want to? What do you think?

Answer: You should do as you prefer, without yielding to pressures either pro or con breast-feeding—and as your doctor thinks best. It certainly can't do your baby any good for you to be unhappy about the way you feed him. And a proper formula will give him everything he needs in the way of nourishment.

Question: I've been told that if I do decide to nurse my baby, I shouldn't eat cabbage. Is this true? I love slaw!

Answer: There isn't any reason to change your diet just because you are nursing—that is, unless your baby seems to object to something you've eaten. One warning, however: don't take any strong laxatives, or you'll give your baby diarrhea!

Question: My doctor suggests that I feed the baby whenever she seems to want food. Why? Wouldn't a schedule be easier?

Answer: Newborns should eat within a very short time after hunger pangs start. Waiting too long for food is an extremely uncomfortable experience, not to mention the fact that crying will tire your baby, so that the edge is taken off her appetite and she is apt to drift off to sleep before she really gets enough to eat. Your baby's contentment and well-being are really the aim of self-demand or self-regulated feeding. Listen to your doctor. And I'm sure you'll find that the baby will want food at fairly regular intervals, so there you'll have your schedule, after all.

Question: Yes, but what do I do if my baby wants food every half hour or so? And sometimes she does! Is this right? When she keeps it up around the clock, I'm so groggy that I hardly know what I'm doing!

Answer: This does happen sometimes. After the first few days, when baby is often too sleepy to eat, she may start eating, as you mention, around the clock. However, she *will* develop her own schedule. To guide her toward eating at regular intervals, you might try other things when you know she has eaten quite recently. For instance, you might try changing her position. Or she may need a change of diapers, not food at all! Rock her for a little while. Then if she keeps on crying, she is probably hungry. Always be sure to give her all that she wants to eat—a full baby is a sleepy baby.

Question: My baby seems to spit up so much milk. Why is this? He's the picture of health, but he *does* spit up!

Answer: If you'd measure the amount of milk (not easy, but if you could measure it!) you'd probably discover that the amount of milk he spits up over a twenty-four-hour period isn't more than half of one feeding. It just seems like lots when you clean it up. But the cause? Doctors used to think it was because the milk didn't agree with the baby. However, now most of them feel that in most cases only *time* can help the baby who spits up. His digestive system is still new, after all, and in need of practice.

Question: Why is my new baby so much harder to burp than his older brother and sister were?

Answer: Somehow one baby simply takes longer to get up a bubble than others do. You might try pushing your baby's tummy firmly against your shoulder while you rub his back. Or why not try comforting him or playing with him (quietly!) for a little while before you start to burp him? If nothing works, just put him down on his stomach. Sooner or later the bubble comes up.

Question: Is it all right for a baby to be on his stomach? I keep worrying—mightn't he smother?

Answer: In spite of old wives' tales, most doctors now agree that it is perfectly safe for a baby to be on its tummy. Even before a baby can hold his head erect, he can turn it from side to side for air. Of course you'll want to take such precautions as being sure the sheet is taut under him—and don't use a pillow.

Question: When I bathe my baby, should I wash out her eyes and mouth?

Answer: Nature does its own cleaning job on a baby's eyes and mouth. You can wipe off your baby's eyelids with a moistened cotton puff, but no other cleansing is necessary.

Question: Is it all right to wash the soft spots on my baby's head? She's so tiny and delicate, I'm afraid I'll damage her!

Answer: Don't worry, she's hardier than she seems—and those soft spots, or fontanels, are tougher than they feel. Actually, the best way to prevent "cradle cap" is to wash the baby's head regularly. Be sure that you rinse it well, too, and of course dry it thoroughly.

Question: Sometimes my baby jumps as if she is startled. Why? Is this normal?

Answer: It's not only normal, it's a sort of "mass reflex" which all new babies should have. Actually, babies do respond more to actual noise. This reflex disappears in three or four months. And in the meantime you needn't keep quiet as a mouse for the baby's sake. Just go on about your normal routine.

Question: My baby seems to wheeze a lot and breathe noisily! I'm not really worried, for the doctor says he's in fine health, but I keep wondering why it is, and I'm afraid the doctor will think I'm one of these superanxious mothers if I keep asking him. So could you tell me?

Answer: In brand-new babies, this may be due to some mucus left in the breathing apparatus from prebirth days. This does make them wheeze a bit for a few days, but it clears up. Some babies do keep on wheezing and "snoring" some, until their nervous systems take firmer control of their breathing. Swallowed bubbles may also make a baby breathe noisily.

Question: It worries me when my baby spits up, but I've been told that spitting up isn't the same as vomiting. Is this true?

Answer: Yes, there is a difference between vomiting and spitting up. Spitting up usually follows feeding and is nothing to worry about, while vomiting is much more severe and can be caused by illness, an infection or a stomach irritation, and often needs medical attention.

Question: Precisely what is diarrhea? What is the difference between it and normal bowel movements?

Answer: In diarrhea, the bowel movements are frequent and fluid, with varying color and odor. In infants, diarrhea is seldom related to food; it is more frequently caused by infection, either in the bowel or elsewhere in the body. Persistent diarrhea should be reported to the doctor at once, as it can cause dehydration and even death.

Question: My mother worries if my little one doesn't have at least one bowel movement every day; yet the doctor isn't at all upset over it. I trust him very much, but I respect my mother's experience, too, and don't know whom to believe!

Answer: Each baby, as your doctor knows, has an individual nervous system and a tendency for the bowel to regulate its own performance. The idea that a baby *must* have one or two movements each and every day is no longer accepted. Some youngsters will have two or three each day, others only one, while still others—equally normal and healthy—will have them only every other day. It isn't abnormal unless it is a definite change from an established pattern. Constipation in babies is not nearly the problem it was before baby foods became widely used. It is highly unlikely to exist if a reasonable variety and amount of supplementary foods are served. Commercially prepared baby foods have thus not only contributed to mother's convenience, but in a significant way to baby's contentment and improved bowel regularity.

Question: Is it really a bad habit for a baby to suck its thumb?
Answer: That's another matter which has apparently come full circle. All children suck their thumbs or fingers (sometimes toes!) at some time during the first five years of life, and young babies who suck thumbs are often the most contented. The idea that this was a "bad habit" didn't appear until the end of the nineteenth century, when alarmists claimed that thumb-sucking caused colic, enlarged tonsils, adenoids and tooth decay. Attempts to stop thumb-sucking often do more harm than good—substituting blanket sucking, facial tics or sometimes behavioral disturbances. When left alone, most children have completely stopped sucking by the age of five years.

Question: Does teething cause illness? Some people have told me it does, others that, of course, it doesn't. What do you say?
Answer: Well, the gum over an erupting tooth can become irritated and inflamed and cause considerable discomfort. However, just because the baby is teething, don't attribute all problems to that—a runny nose and a cold, for instance, just happen to occur at the same time. They are not caused by the teething itself.

Question: I believe in children having plenty of fresh air and sunshine, but of course I don't want to overdo it. About how long may I leave my baby outside?
Answer: Always remember to time sunbathing carefully. To start out, only a minute or so; then add a minute a day, up

to a maximum of fifteen minutes, front and back. You really shouldn't sun a baby between the hours of 10 A.M. and 2 P.M., or on very hot days, and it's a good idea to protect baby's eyes by placing the crown of the head toward the sun. Also, if you take your baby to the beach, cut the time to half, even if it is an overcast, cloudy day.

Question: My baby has swollen breasts. I was afraid I had given birth to a freak, until I discovered some other cases of this—some girls say their babies' breasts even contained "milk." Is this possible? What causes it? What should be done for it?

Answer: These swollen breasts and fluid—not really milk—are due to hormones from the mother's body. They may be found in both boy and girl babies. Just leave them alone. Don't handle the breasts, and you'll find that they will soon return to normal.

Question: Is it just my imagination, or did my youngster's temper improve after he learned to talk?

Answer: It probably wasn't your imagination. Being unable to communicate is quite a source of frustration, so it stands to reason that as children learn to talk, to make plain what they want, what they like and dislike, they are less frustrated and accordingly are sunnier-tempered.

Question: How long should I expect my baby to wear diapers?

Answer: The average baby will need diapers full-time for at least a year, and will keep on wearing them part-time for another six months to a year. It would be nice if babies would toilet-train earlier, but they simply aren't physically able, so there's no point in trying to force them.

Question: I've noticed some children's clothing and so on are labeled "fire-retardant." Is that the same as "fireproof"?

Answer: No, not quite. Fire-retardant means that the material has been treated so that if it does catch fire, it will smolder slowly—giving you time to put out the fire before serious injury is incurred—rather than burning with a blaze. You can make your own fire-retardant solution and treat clothing, etc., by mixing 7 ounces borax, 3 ounces boric acid and 2 quarts of hot water. Dip items into the solution and press with a warm, not hot, iron.

Question: My little boy hurt his lip. I knew that putting ice

on it would help, but he wouldn't let me. Boys being boys, this may happen again, so I'm wondering if you have any ideas how to persuade him to go along with the ice treatment?
Answer: You might try outsmarting him—let him eat a popsicle. It will take his mind off the hurt lip, and the popsicle *is* ice, after all. The pain and swelling should be gone by the time the popsicle is consumed.

Question: We plan to go to my parents' home—two hundred miles away—for Christmas, and I'm wondering what would be the best way to dress the baby, especially while traveling?
Answer: A good choice would be all-in-one-piece stretch suits or leotard suits. They're comfortable for the baby both night and day, protect against chilling and are neat. Also, you can easily add bonnets, sweaters and shawls if chilly, and they're ideal under pram suits as well—not bulky, as nightgowns can be.

Question: What would be the best solution to the diaper problem while we're traveling and visiting? We'll be away a week. I'd rather not do diapers the whole time we're visiting, and a supply large enough to last without washing would be too bulky to pack.
Answer: This would be a good time for you to use either disposable diapers or disposable diaper liners. You might also check into the possibility of having diaper service while there. If you use a diaper service at home, talk to them—the company may offer vacation service or be able to recommend a service at your destination.

Question: Do babies get carsick? What should I do if mine does?
Answer: Babies under the age of nine months seldom get carsick. In fact, most babies seem to enjoy traveling. Carsickness seems to run in families, so if other members of your family are susceptible, you can be prepared, just in case, with an older baby. Your doctor might give you an antinauseant, but cutting out milk is a good preventive. So is feeding only light meals or letting the youngster nibble dry crackers.

Question: We love to camp and think we've figured out most of the problems of taking the baby along, but we wonder about bathing him, since sometimes there's just a limited amount of water.

Answer: As long as you keep the diaper area scrupulously clean, your baby won't suffer. You can keep his face, hands, etc., clean with packaged, ready-dampened washcloths.

Question: I think my baby intends to grow up to be a nudist. How he hates to be dressed or to have his clothes changed! Have you any suggestions?

Answer: If you can distract his attention, you've got the battle half won. Try giving him a toy *before* you start dressing him, so that it absorbs his attention while you do a quick change job. He'll eventually resign himself to the inevitable.

Question: My youngster doesn't mind getting dressed at all, but can he ever strip fast! Then he heads for the great outdoors. What shall I do? We're new in the neighborhood, and what must the neighbors think of us!

Answer: For one thing, keep the screen door hooked. That will at least keep him indoors. You might make a point of dressing him in clothes which fasten up the back—less easy for him to remove!—until he outgrows this phase. And be comforted—this is not a very prudish age, and most people know that very small children are inclined this way and are amused, not horrified. Your neighbors doubtless understand.

Question: I know children's feet grow fast and they shouldn't wear shoes which are outgrown, but how can I tell when the shoes are too small?

Answer: You're right, little ones do outgrow their shoes quite rapidly, making it a good idea to check fit at frequent intervals. Some signs that new shoes are in order are tightness across the instep and the toes—no growing room left at the toes—and wrinkled leather, bulging sides and sagging heels. Feet grow—shoes don't.

Question: I keep worrying when people hold my baby. It isn't that I don't trust them, but he isn't exactly housebroken yet! I'd hate for them to have drenched laps. They'd understand, of course, but even so, how can I prevent it?

Answer: This is one of the occasions when Gerber baby pants come in very handy. They're made of a sturdy polyvinyl film which is waterproof, leakproof and acidproof. And, where your baby himself is concerned, we've made sure

QUESTIONS MANY MOTHERS ASK

that our Gerber baby pants won't stiffen up—they'll stay soft—and they're bound in a dainty nylon edging for soft contact with a baby's little legs and waist. They're amply cut to allow wiggling room and room to grow, come in three sizes, in both pull-on and snap-on styles *and* they're machine-washable, made to last through many launderings. We're pretty proud of them.

Question: My little girl likes to dress herself, but she has some trouble getting her shoes on the proper feet. How can I teach her which is which?

Answer: Several mothers have shared their solutions to this problem with me, so I'll pass them on—take your pick! They drew things in the shoes—the simplest was arrows pointing at each other; or hands with fingers pointing at each other. Still another was a face in each shoe—when the shoes were right to put on the proper feet, the profiles were smiling at one another. This not only helps a child get shoes on the proper feet, but makes doing so fun!

Question: How can I keep a film from forming on the inside of my baby's bottles and nipples?

Answer: Start by rinsing your bottles, nipples and formula pans in cold water right after emptying them. Then fill them with warm water (the addition of a water softener helps) and soak until you're ready to wash them. When you do wash them, use hot water and scrub with a stiff bottle brush. Turn the nipples inside out to be sure you clean them completely. Rinse them well, then sterilize the bottles and nipples before you refill them.

Question: This question isn't about my baby, exactly—I haven't had it yet. I'm wondering what I should pack to take to the hospital when I have the baby.

Answer: You'll need nightgowns, a robe and slippers (flat-heeled), your cosmetics, brush and comb, plus a mirror. Toothbrush and toothpaste and deodorant. It's also a good idea to take along note paper and stamps so that you can write and tell people about that wonderful baby! Sanitary belt. Cleansing tissues. You might take along some small change, too, for newspaper, etc. Most hospitals have gift shops. If you like to read, you might take along paperback books or magazines (I've found that small, digest-sized magazines are easier to read in bed than large ones). You might keep your packed bag in the car to make sure it isn't forgotten in the excitement or blocking the door at night so that you can't possibly leave without it. And while you are packing, you might want to include your "coming-home" clothes so that your husband won't have to rummage around assembling them to bring to you.

Question: What about scales? Should I have them and weigh the baby at any special times?

Answer: Your doctor will weigh your baby during regular checkups. If you get scales, weighing baby once a week is often enough. Babies' weights have their ups and downs, and when a baby is weighed daily, it's easy to fret about the loss of an ounce or so.

Question: I've heard there's a difference between the way you put diapers on boy babies and girl babies. What is it?

Answer: In diapering a baby boy, you place the thickest folds of the diaper in front. In diapering a little girl, the thickest part goes in back.

Question: I know there are special cereals for babies, but wouldn't regular adult cereals be just as good?

Answer: Not really. Gerber cereals, at least, are enriched with iron, calcium and B vitamins. And they're tasty enough that often adults prefer them, too (they may give mother just that little needed boost to cope with a lively youngster!).

Question: Is the "Gerber baby" a real baby? Is it a boy or a girl? Is it one of your children or grandchildren?

Answer: No, it is not. It's a sketch of a model whose identity is a Gerber secret. It's a sketch done by artist Dorothy Hope Smith, which charmed us all so much that it became our trademark. I think it looks like a little girl, but other people are just as positive it's a boy. She was simply creating the most adorable baby possible!

Appendix

Why Throw Them Away?

This section is not directed to you as a mother but as both a thrifty and creative person who—like myself, for one—hates to throw away those perfectly good baby food containers. Now obviously you can't reuse all those baby food jars to keep leftovers, dibs of this, dabs of that. What do others find to do with them? You'd be surprised!

Ever think of painting the lids, then filling the jars with herbs and spices? Most variety stores have stick-on labels which you can apply to the jars to identify the contents, or you might decorate the jars and their lids with painted designs.

THE USES OF BABY FOOD JARS

Baby food jars are just fine for storing little things like coconut, chocolate chips, nutmeats and so on, after the packages have been opened—especially if the original was a cellophane or plastic bag which keeps tearing or opening and spilling contents all through the cupboard.

Baby food jars are also great for carrying just the right amount of bleach and detergent when you go to the laundromat. Or fill one with water softener.

Fathers have been quick to latch on to the baby food jars their offspring empty, and the things they do with them!

Tacks, assorted nails, screws and other workshop items can be kept separated and orderly when each item is put in its own Gerber jar. If the jar tops are nailed onto the bottom of a shelf the jars can be twisted on and off in a jiffy.

Leftover paint keeps in them very nicely for a long time. It'll be right there, handy for touch-ups, with the paint's color showing through the clear glass jar: no need to open can after can of paint to find the shade you want.

One enterprising couple built a low garden wall, or a planter, using emptied Gerber jars. They put colored artificial flowers in some of the jars to add eye appeal.

Sports-minded parents have found baby food jars to be just the thing for storing small things such as golf tees, fish hooks and artificial bait.

Like to garden? How about using baby food jars to store seeds or to start cuttings? Or you might put seed packets in them, at the end of rows, to identify which seeds were planted in those rows.

Jars come in handy when encouraging your youngsters to develop an interest in gardening. Children love to start planting such things as grapefruit, orange and lemon seeds, or carrot tops. Or you might fill the jars with pebbles for starting your Easter bulbs.

INFINITE VARIETY

In the feminine equivalent of a man's workshop you might sort pins, snaps, buttons, needles, thimbles, hooks, etc., into their own jars to save pawing through a mass of sewing equipment (and invariably stabbing your finger on a needle or pin). If you embroider, you might put each color of embroidery thread into a separate jar. That keeps it clean as well as organized.

Emptied baby food jars are equally useful as desk organizers. Store paper clips, stamps and rubber bands in them. A small ball of string in a jar with one end extending through a hole in the lid is very convenient. Other jars can be used as holders for pens, pencils, erasers and crayons. You might also keep Christmas tags and stickers in the jars.

Hobbies! The ways in which hobbyists use empty Gerber jars are far too numerous to name, and brand-new hobby uses crop up in every day's mail. Here are just a few of them:

APPENDIX 187

* Gerber baby food jars are used in schoolrooms for paint and paste jars and for cleaning paint brushes, too.
* Ceramicists use them for storing paints and finishes for their ceramic projects.
* Photographers think they're just the thing in darkrooms to store small rolls of film that have been developed, plus other little items such as rubber bands, art gum, clips and labels.
* Stamp and coin collectors favor baby food jars for sorting and storing their collections until transferring them to books and albums.
* Rock hounds can store their finds in the jars—baby food jars are ideal for showing off agates and other small specimens in water.
* Small shells, gems, beads, tweezers and "findings" for jewelry making can be kept neatly sorted out in jars.

Some laboratories use baby food jars to store small equipment and as specimen jars.

Baby food jars come in handy in the bathroom, too (up high enough that toddlers can't get into them when exploring). You can use them for storing hairpins, vitamins, aspirin, hairnets, powder puffs, rolls of gauze, cotton puffs, Band-Aids and so on.

In the nursery (very appropriate, since after all the jars were originally purchased for baby), you can use the jars to store pins, cotton puffs and various other little items.

Baby food jars make good little banks, too.

They're just great on picnics—they're convenient disposable containers for such things as sugar, cream (or powdered cream substitute), mustard, ketchup, sauces, pickles. They make fine outdoor ashtrays, too. You might put baby's cereal into a jar at home and take it along to be mixed with formula when it's time to feed baby. (This is an idea for your traveling, too.) Instant coffee and tea bags also keep quite well in them.

BEING CREATIVE WITH JARS

Groups, such as the Boy Scouts and the Girl Scouts, have decorated baby food jars and filled them with such things as homemade candy samples, fresh flowers or artificial flowers. These have been used as gifts for children in hospitals and for neighborhood shut-ins, to say nothing of Mother's Day and Father's Day gifts.

Jars have also been filled with rose petals, pine needles and sachet bags to make attractive, convenient little fragrance jars for closets and dresser drawers.

Gerber baby food jars have been decorated with sequins, crepe paper, ribbons, lace, paint, yarn and raffia. They've been filled with pebbles or sand to hold flowers in place. Decorated, they've been used as nut cups, favors and candle holders. A variety of homemade toppings for ice cream sundaes may be stored in the jars and served from them.

Speaking of candle holders, it's amazing what handsome and impressive ones can be made from several Gerber jars fastened together and gilded, painted or antiqued. They look really gorgeous.

Many creative people have made delightful special-occasion gifts from empty Gerber baby food jars. They've arranged plastic flowers upside down in a water-filled jar, capped it (very securely, mind, if you try it) then turned it upside down for a paperweight.

Just one word of caution: strange as it may seem, inasmuch as baby food jars were originally used for canned foods, reusing them for home canning is *not* recommended. The reason for this is that the jar lids were designed for a single use only, and for applications under precise conditions of temperature, pressure and torque which cannot be duplicated at home. An airtight seal can't be assured when you reuse the lids, applying them by hand.

Probably you'll be thinking of additional uses for Gerber baby food jars. Let us know. We are always interested in hearing the new uses which you find. Even those jars that are discarded are likely to be recycled into useful purposes. This is especially true when they are discarded through a city disposal system in which sorting is economically feasible.

Index

American Academy of Family
  Physicians, 9
Apple juice, 41
Apricot Surprise Pudding, 169
Art, use in nursery, 18
Artificial respiration, 156–157

Baby bath, 17
"Baby caddy," 19
Baby sitters,
  daytime, 109–111
  health of, 113
  information for, 104–107, 108
  interviewing, 101–102
  payment for, 107
  preparing baby for, 107
  rules for, 103–104
  teen-agers as, 105–107
  to find, 100–101
Baked goods, 50–51
Bath-time ideas
  plastic wallpaper, 63
  surfer's watch, 63
  use of spice rack, 63
  use of water conditioner, 63
Bassinet, 16

Bathing, 58–63
  "real" bath, 59–61
  care of rash, 62
  drying, 63
  fingernails, 62
  fun time, 61
  nose, 62
  order of bath, 60
  preparation for, 60
  removing from tub, 62–63
  shampoo, 60–61
  washing ears, 61
  water temperature, 60
  sponge baths, 59
Bathing equipment, 12
Bedspread, for bassinet, 18
Beet Borsch, 168
Behavior, acceptable and
  unacceptable, 116
Bellyband, 173
Birth
  length, 25
  weight, 25
Bites
  animal, 158

INDEX

insect, 158
snake, 157–158
Blackboard, 19
Blankets, 67
Blocks, 140–141
Booster shots, 159
Bottle feeding, 33
  position, 33
Bowel movements, 178–179
Bowlegs, 174
Breast-feeding, 33, 175–176
Bruises, 154–155
Bubbling, 177
Burns
  chemical, 155
  extensive, 155
  minor, 155
Bus travel, 165–166

Cabbage, while nursing, 176
Calcium, 44
Car bed, place for, 163
Carrot-and-Cheese Soufflé, 168
Carsickness, 181
Cereals, 43–44, 184
Choking, 156
Clinging to objects, 127
Clothing
  amount, 67
  fire retardant, 180
  hot weather, 175
  while traveling, 181
Clothing list, 11
  quality, 13
    to test, 13
Combinations, vegetables and meat, 48
Comparisons, 144–145
Competition with child, parental, 144
Consistency, 117–118, 121
Constancy, 117–118
Cottage cheese, 49
Cradle cap, 177
Crawling, 26, 81–82
Crayons, 142–143
Cream of Vegetable Soup, 168
Creativity, 135–136
Crib, when traveling, 164
Crying, 71–73
  reasons for, 72–73
Cup, drinking from, 49
Custards, 53
Cuts, 155

Daily food plan, 38
  bread-cereal group, 38
  meat group, 38
  milk group, 38
  vegetable-fruit group, 38
Desserts, 53
Diapering, 184
Diapers, 63–64, 175
  disposable, 161, 181
Diaper service, 63
Diarrhea, 178
Discipline, 114–116, 121
Doctor, when to call, 153–158

Eating schedule, 176
Egg yolks, 46
Extra hair ("lanugo"), 173
Eyes
  chemicals in, 156
  foreign bodies in, 156

Fainting, 156
Falling, 83–84, 94
Feeding problems, 55–57
  mealtime discipline, 57
Film on bottles and nipples, 183
Finger foods, 54
Finger marks, removing, 19
Fingernail care, 62
Fontanel, 26
Food
  storing at home, 55
  warming, 162–163
  when traveling, 162–163
Food plan, 38
Formulas, 33
  when traveling, 161–162
Fractures, 155
Fresh air, 67–69, 179–180
Fruits, 46–48
Fruit-Salad Dressing, 169
Frustration, 130–132
Furniture, renovating, 17

Going home, 27–28
Grow-chart, 20

Harmful play, 147
Head injuries, 156
Head shape, 173
Hearing, 77–78
Help, at home, 32
High meat dinners, 48–49

INDEX

Immunization, 158–159
  D.T.P. (diphtheria, tetanus, pertussis), 159
  polio, 159
  smallpox, 159
Instructional materials, 134
Iron, 44

Japanese wind chimes, 19
Junior foods, 54

Lagging appetite, 52
Laundry, 64–66
  delicate fabrics, 64–65
  hand-washing, 65
  plastic pants, 65
  stains, 65
  sweaters, 65
  toys, 65
  water temperature, 64
Laxatives, while nursing, 176
Left-handedness, 80–81
Listening, 141–142
Lullabies, 78–79

"Mass reflex," 177–178
Mealtime, 36
  dawdling, 52–53
  equipment, 11
  schedules, 37
  tips, 53
Meat, 44–46
  vitamins in, 45
Menu planning, 49–50
Milk, 38–39, 40
Milk rebellion, 51–52
Mock Chicken Legs, 169
Mother substitute, 111–113

Name, selecting, 20
Navel "pop out," 174
Needs and wants, differences between, 116, 119–121
  guidelines, 120–121
"Normal new-baby jaundice," 174
Nosebleeds, 156
Nose, cleaning, 62
Nursery, 14–17
  basics, 15
  equipment, 12
  lack of space, 15
Obstetrician, selecting, 9

Orange juice, 41
  from cup, 49
Organization, 32–33
Outing equipment, 12
Overalls, 14
Overcontrol, 119

Packing, 164
Pasta, 50
Pediatrician, selecting, 28
  questions for, 29
Pegboard, use of, 18–19
Pets, 147–148
Phosphorus, 44
Picture books, storing, 19
Plane travel, 165–166
Planning ahead, 21–22
  getting to hospital, 23
  packing for hospital, 22, 183–184
Plastic bags, 95
Plastic dishes, 95
Plastic nursers, 161
Plastic tablecloth, when traveling, 165
Play area, when traveling, 163
Playpen, 136–138
  tips for, 138–139
  when traveling, 164
Playthings and/or play interests, lists
  one month to eight months, 149
  six months to one year, 149
  one year to eighteen months, 149–150
  eighteen months to two years, 150
  two to two-and-a-half years, 150
Playtime, regulating, 145–147
Poison
  fumes or gases, 157
  in the eye, 157
  on the skin, 157
  swallowed, 157
"Port-wine stains," 174
Potatoes, 50
Pudding, 53
Pulling up, 81
Puncture wounds, 155

Rag dolls, 14
Rash, 174–175
  care of, 62
  diaper, 175

INDEX

Rate of development, 79–81
Rate of growth, 25
Responding to faces, 75–77
  crying, 77
  smiling, 75–76
Restaurants, when traveling, 165
Rhythmic movements, 127
Rolling over, 81
Room temperature, 66

Safety, 87–97
  automobiles
    car bed, 95
    car seat, 95
  bathtub, 87–88
  crib, 87
  hazards, indoors, 88–93
    bedroom, 91
    dangers, 92
    high chair, 89
    kitchen, 89–90, 92
    medicine, 91
    stairs, 89
    windows, 89
  hazards, outdoors, 93–94
    animals, 93–94
    insecticide, 93
    pesticide, 93
    power tools, 93
Safety checklist, 95–97
  in basement or garage, 97
  in bathroom, 97
  in bedroom, 97
  in general, 96
  in kitchen, 96
  in yard, 97
Scales, 184
Scrapbook, 29
Scrapes, 154
Seeing, 75–76
  focusing, 75
Self-discipline, parental, 122–123
Self-feeding, 51
Sharing, 143–144
Shoes, 183
  putting on, 183
Shopping, 10–11, 12
  for nursery, 15
Sitting, 26, 81
Sleep, 29–31
  how much, 30, 69–71
  noise and, 31
  position, 31

Sleeping bags, 67
Slivers, 155
Smiling, 26, 34, 75–76
Socks, 13
Solids, first, 41–43
  how to feed, 42–43
  position, 42
Spicy Applesauce Molds, 169
Spitting up, 176–177, 178
Spoiling, 13
Sprains, 156
Standing, 82
Stroller, when traveling, 164
Sucking, 34
Sunshine, 68–69
Swollen breasts, baby, 180

Talking, 84–85
Talking to baby, 84–85
Teething, 26, 179
Teething biscuits, 50
Telephone numbers, list for posting, 152
Temper tantrums, 129–130
"The Ice Game," 142
Thiamine, 44
Threats, 118–119
Thumb-sucking, 124–127, 179
Toilet seat, when traveling, 165
Toilet training, 128–129
Toys, 137, 139–140
Toys, when traveling, 164
Train travel, 165–166
Tuberculosis test, 159

Undercontrol, 119

Veal Mousse, 169
Vegetables, 46–48
  green, 48
  yellow, 47
Vitamin C, 41
Vitamins, 40

Walking, 26, 83–84
Wastebasket, 17
Water, 40
  from cup, 49
  when traveling, 163
Waterproof pants, 13
Wheezing, 178
Window shades, 18

Zwieback, 50